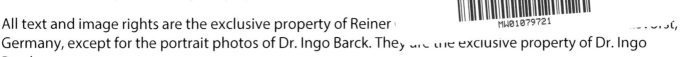

1st Edition 2016

Pictures of all Arm Chair exercises: Photographer Miriam Abels; info@mimmoi.de

All texts: Reiner Grootenhuis, assisted by Dr. Ingo Barck in the chapter "Everything you need to know about the Arm Chair", in all exercise descriptions in the section "Aims of the exercise" and in the "Glossary"

Model: Carla Sophie Nacken (and Reiner Grootenhuis in the chapter "Assistance")

Photo shoot assistant: Felicitas Ruthe

Translation from German: lengoo GmbH, Erbprinzenstr. 29a, D-76133 Karlsruhe

ISBN-13: 978-1537486888

ISBN-10: 1537486888

Contact information of the authors:

Reiner Grootenhuis

Email: info@pilates-powers.de

Phone: 0157 / 340 340 40

Website: http://www.pilates-powers.de

Dr. Ingo Barck

Email: ingo@dr-barck.de

Phone: 02152 - 95 99 0 99

Website: http://www.dr-barck.de/

Table of contents

Preface Reiner Grootenhuis

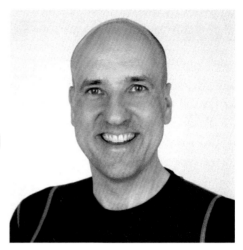

Nowadays, the Arm Chair as a piece of Pilates equipment has nearly been forgotten about and hardly any Pilates studio has one. While training on a mat and with the Reformer is very popular now, and working with a Cadillac/Tower and the Wunda Chair is being offered more often, the Pilates Arm Chair is sadly not widely known. Thus, the knowledge about the Arm Chair is very limited as well. Let me put this in numbers:

One of the best-known Pilates video platforms worldwide, Pilates Anytime, offers Pilates videos with Pilates workshops and classes. Most of its clients are Pilates instructors that use the platform to educate themselves further. As the video platform is very successful and enjoys high acceptance, one can assume that the information offered on the website coincides with the interests of the Pilates instructors. In March 20151, the video platform Pilates Anytime offered 1,093 videos for mat workouts, 440 Reformer classes and workshops, 115 Cadillac plus 54 Tower videos, as well as 104 Wunda Chair videos - to name but a few.[1]

There are only 4 videos about the Arm Chair. This is a mere 0.2 % from 1,917 available Pilates videos.

With this manual, my goal is to contribute to a greater spread and use of this fantastic piece of Pilates equipment.

To be honest, I, too, was unsure for quite some time whether I should buy an Arm Chair for my studio or not. Although I had already been acquainted with a modern form of the Arm Chair during my BASI© Pilates studio education, I thought that I could perform the exercises I had learnt with my light arm springs and a Reformer Sitting Box as well. Back then, I was not aware of the importance of the support of the back and especially of the feedback of the chair for the shoulders given by the backrest on the "traditional" Arm Chair.

Today, I am very happy that I chose to get a "traditional" Arm Chair as it is the perfect addition for training with my private clients. The Arm Chair is incredibly versatile and especially helpful when working out with people that have shoulder or neck problems.

It would be a great pleasure to me if you shared my enthusiasm for the Arm Chair after reading this training manual.

Tönisvorst, March 2016   Reiner Grootenhuis

---

[1] Accessed March 17th, 2016, 3:23 pm

Preface Dr. Ingo Barck

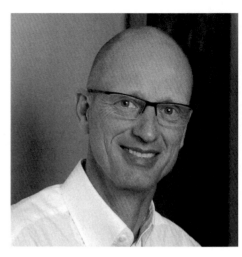

In the course of my work as a sports physician and especially during the manual therapeutic diagnosis of patients suffering from pain, I have observed muscle contractures and muscular imbalances over and over again. Many have already performed intensive training with training devices but have noticed no significant improvement of their symptoms. This is typical as only few regard coordinative abilities and mobility during their workouts. Most people believe in cardio or strength training being a cure. In reality, however, this does not remove the causes of most pains.

These namely arise from deficits in coordination, muscular imbalances and contractures, which result from prolonged sitting.

I met Reiner Grootenhuis amongst a group of entrepreneurs and he introduced me to the Pilates method. My enthusiasm for Pilates was aroused pretty quickly since it was obvious that this form of training was able to remove the deficits mentioned above. Not only can it help many patients suffering from pain but also prevent pain from occurring at all.

The complexity of Pilates exercises always includes a coordinative task that engages many different muscles or muscle groups. Furthermore, it promotes the mobility of the musculoskeletal system.

The special myofascial release therapy has also been incorporated into the concept of Pilates. Thus, Pilates is a very complex form of training that regards the muscular and fascial system and all its specific needs.

Despite its simple construction, the Arm Chair offers multiple training possibilities. It is also suitable for those with physical limitations due to its low spring resistance, so that they can work out without excessive demand.

Kempen, March 2016 Dr. Ingo Barck

Preface Carla Sophie

My name is Carla Sophie, I am 20 years old and have been doing Pilates at the pilates-powers studio for nearly 3.5 years now. I work out in different areas (mat, Tower, Wunda Chair) 2-3 times a week. When I started doing this previously unknown sport in the fall of 2012, I originally just wanted to try something new. I had always been athletic: whether it was tennis, ballet, running, swimming, or soccer, I had tried almost every sport.

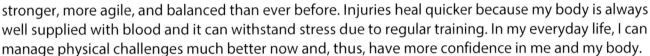

Today I can say with 100% certainty: I never want to live without Pilates again. In the past 3 years, my body has undergone such immense development, I would never have thought it possible. I am stronger, more agile, and balanced than ever before. Injuries heal quicker because my body is always well supplied with blood and it can withstand stress due to regular training. In my everyday life, I can manage physical challenges much better now and, thus, have more confidence in me and my body.

Even after all this time, I learn about new exercises and variations during my workouts and am amazed over and over again at how versatile Pilates is. This is also the reason why I am still so enthusiastic about it and why it is the only thing that I have kept pursuing the past few years. It is never boring since the range of exercises is so wide and new things are constantly added.

Due to a genetic malposition of my wrists, my range of motion in these joints is rather limited. Thanks to personalized exercises, which slowly but surely allowed me to test the full potential of my wrists, I have gained improved stability in these joints so that they can withstand more and especially longer periods of stress. Even limitations like these cannot hold you back in Pilates.

However, the many workouts have not only improved my muscles, joints and mobility, but Pilates has given me something else that I never would have thought possible: with a height of only 154 cm, I was always the smallest person. Even though I had learned to live with this over the years, I was excited beyond words when I had my measurements professionally taken by my doctor recently - 158 cm. My posture has improved during this time so much that I gained 4 cm in height. All of this is why I can only say: Pilates makes dreams come true!

Krefeld, March 2016 Carla Sophie

Pilates, a training guided by principles

Pilates is special. There are only a few forms of movement that unite movement and concentration in a similar way.

Over the course of his life, Joseph Pilates developed equipment and exercises, which he always adapted to his clients' needs. He had a clear idea of how his exercises were to be performed. With the help of co-authors, he tried to explain the broader context of his musculoskeletal system "Contrology", as he called it, in three publications. Sadly, this often ended on the level of advertisement for his system. At the studio, he was rather taciturn as well and, as Joseph Pilates' lawyer and client John Steele stated in an interview[1], he was someone who merely said "no" without explaining how to improve the exercise. Verbalizing all his findings and knowledge is reserved for his students.

For example, Joseph Pilates did not use the term principles. This means that the so-called Pilates principles are something that was added later or was extracted from the method. The first to use the term Pilates principles were Philip Friedman and Gail Eisen. Both had been students of Romana Kryzanowska. In 1980, they published the first book on Pilates: "The Pilates Method of Physical and Mental Conditioning." According to their own statement, Romana Kryzanowska more or less dictated the book to Philip Friedman and Gail Eisen. The same six principles were later published again in "The Pilates Method of Body Conditioning" by Sean P. Gallagher & Romana Kryzanowska (1999). The six principles are:

1. Concentration
2. Centering
3. Control
4. Breathing
5. Precision
6. Flowing movement

My personal interpretation of the six principles is:

Concentration

Joseph Pilates said: "Contrology is complete coordination of body, mind, and spirit."[2] In order to reach this state, concentration is a crucial condition. This also means that the movements in Pilates are not performed automatically or unconsciously, or that one distracts oneself with television, conversations or music. By concentrating on what one is doing and how one is doing it, one becomes aware of the movement and the processes in the mind during the movement.

Centering

Centering continues the awareness gained by concentration. It is the mental preparation before moving the body, an inner relaxation and an continuous focus on one's inner state. Pilates is no competition. Centering also means preparing the body for the movement that it is about to perform, for example by activating the body's core. This way all movements are performed from a centered mind and body. It is this centering that distinguishes Pilates from similar movements on the mat in other exercise methods.

---

[1] http://www.pilatesanytime.com/workshop-view/2503/video/Pilates-John-Steel-by-John-Steel
[2] Joseph Pilates: „Return to Life through Contrology", (1945), chapter „Contrology restores physical fitness", first sentence

Control

An essential term, as Joseph Pilates called his movement art 'Contrology.' When performing Pilates exercises, nothing is left to chance. One decides to perform an exercise within a certain setup, performs it and continues until the set amount of repetitions is reached. While performing the exercise, one keeps one's body under control as well as the Pilates equipment and its springs. Romana Kryzanowska said: "You can say what Pilates is in these words: Stretch with strength and control. And the control part is the most important because it makes you use your mind".[1]

Breathing

Although Joseph Pilates specified a breathing pattern for each exercise in his book about mat exercises, at the same time his instructions in the studio regarding breathing, were not precise enough to derive a breathing technique from it. Instructors and clients that visited his studio report that he often used "out with the air" as an instruction.[2] Sometimes he also said, "Squeeze out the lungs as you would wring a wet towel dry"[3] So his main idea was to deflate the lungs completely in order to fill them again with fresh air. This was of upmost importance to him and he even designed a device to practice this: the Breath-a-cizer. One can purchase it, for example, at Gratz, a manufacturer of Pilates equipment.

His student Romana Kryzanowska is cited in the book by Philip Friedman and Gail Eisen with the general breathing rule: "Inhale into the tension, exhale when releasing it or relaxing." Or the modification: "If you're doing something that squeezes your body tightly, use the motion to squeeze air out of your lungs and inhale when you straighten up".

In her DVD series "Romana on Pilates: The Legacy Edition," she distinguishes between specific "breathing exercises," i.e. exercises that focus on one's breathing and use a certain breathing pattern, and exercises during which the breath just flows. However, it is certain that one's breath is not held during Pilates and that one exercises a specific control in order to prevent the pressure of the diaphragm from bulging the abdomen outward.

It is proven that our breathing affects the regularity of our heartbeat and, thus, the ability and capacity of our brain. Important: when breathing irregularly, this spreads panic in the body and the brain. It is perceived that there has to be a reason for the irregular breathing. So if one wants to work out in a concentrated and simultaneously attentive manner, finding a regular breathing rhythm is key. The breathing rhythm can adapt to the pattern of movement so that a harmonious connection arises. By the way, the duration of inhaling and exhaling is irrelevant and it does not need to be the same for both parts. The main thing is that the breath stays calm.[4]

People breath and move with a different pace. This also means that the adjustment of breathing and movement is individual. Therefore, I have not included instructions on inhaling and exhaling for every exercise in this manual. Yet on the basis of the information above, I suggest that, after internalizing the movement pattern of every exercise, one should try out breathing patterns for oneself and one's clients and, if useful, use them undogmatically.

[1] Brooke Siler: „The Women'sHealth Big Book of PILATES",(2013)

[2] E.g. http://www.robertwernick.com/articles/pilates.htm; accessed March 26st, 2016, 8:38 pm

[3] Karon Karter: „The Complete Idiot's Guide to the Pilates Method", (2000), in „Chapter 3 Take your Breath"

[4] Alan Watkins: "Being Brilliant Every Single Day" - TEDx Portsmouth http://youtu.be/fRItG9G1rb4 und http://karahpino.me/2013/04/07/b-r-e-a-t-h-e-the-neuroscience-of-breathing-techniques-ted-talk/

Precision

Precise movements are a result of concentration, centering, control and calm breathing. Imagine an archer for whom precision is crucial. Without the qualities mentioned above, he will not hit his target.

Every body is different and, for example, has a different physiognomy while having the same weight. Thus, it is not about making something appear as it does with someone else. Precision applies to one's own performance. If one moves without precision in Pilates, one does not achieve the interaction of the muscle groups, which is the actual goal of the exercise. Therefore, it is important to really understand how to perform the exercises and which goal they pursue. In a next step, one also has to feel this. When performed in this manner, the exercise will be precise.

Flowing movement

Pilates exercises flow. They have a flow within the exercises and, if possible, in the transitions from one exercise to another as well. This way one achieves to keep one's focus during the exercise and the entire workout. If you lose concentration, you lose the flow and have to center yourself in order to continue the exercise. The challenge to keep the flow is greater on or even between equipment than on the mat. Mat exercises are thus well suited to practice keeping the flow of movement through skillful transitions between the exercises.

Addition to the Pilates principles

Already during his youth, Reiner Grootenhuis was introduced to the Chinese movement art Tai Chi. Later he studied the martial art of Weng Chun, which originated from the Southern Shaolin Monastery, under the instruction of grandmaster Andreas Hoffmann. During the ten years of intensive Kung Fu studies, Andreas Hoffmann also taught him the Shaolin Kung Fu Principles of the Shaolin warrior monks.[1] In his experience, these are of importance for studying and teaching Pilates as well: the subjective elements are divided into four elements that one should seek out and three that one should avoid. For Pilates, the three elements that are to be avoided are of special interest.

Avoid TAM - greed

Pilates is a process, a journey. It is not about performing an exercise but about the journey to get there. If I try to do something too quickly that does not fit my place in the journey yet, I will possibly harm myself and suffer a setback on my Pilates journey. The same applies to the expected results. The body will not change overnight but a little bit every day. We do not gain or lose ten kilos in a day and the same goes for other changes in our body - they occur little by little. Wanting too much sets you up for frustration.

Avoid PA - fear

Especially people who have experienced a long period of pain in their lives fear that this pain might recur as well as the helplessness associated with it. Hence, they are often fearful in the beginning when moving and judge a pulling sensation or any kind of discomfort as a sign for the recurring pain. In the long run, the movement of tense and poorly supplied muscle groups causes pain relief and prevention.

Yet, fear does not only occur with patients suffering from pain. The more advanced the exercises become, the more they appear like a circus performance. It can then happen quickly that one experiences fear. It is important to understand that one's own Pilates performance benefits from facing one's fears over and over again without wanting too much all at once.

---

[1]Andreas Hoffmann: "Weng Chun Kung Fu - Die weiche Kraft von Shaolin", (2002), p. 41

Avoid MONG - confusion

When performing the exercises, some people have problems remembering the sequence of the more complex exercises like Boomerang and Rowing. In this moment, confusion arises and disrupts the exercise flow. In cases like these, it is important to break down the exercise to a simple part of the exercise in order to overcome the confusion as quickly as possible.

It is also possible that one feels overwhelmed while studying and practicing due to the large amount of exercises and many adjustment possibilities of the equipment. The better one's understanding of the system is, the clearer it becomes that all exercises are tightly related to each other and that often an exercise is "merely" another possibility for training one aspect or feeling. In moments of confusion, it is thus advisable to look for a related exercise that one knows well and to remember the feelings and movements one has experienced during this exercise. This newly gained focus makes starting the next exercise much easier.

Everything you need to know about the Arm Chair

The Arm Chair is also called Baby Chair. This is probably because its springs are the lightest springs in a traditional studio, which are also sometimes called Baby Arm Springs or Baby Springs.

Not much is known about the origin of the Baby Chair. Yet, it is certain that it was already in use in Joseph Pilates' studio, according to Esperanza Aparicio & Javier Pérez' biography "Hubertus Joseph Pilates – The Biography."[1] They report that Joseph Pilates tried to record his work towards the end of his life and created a series of 12 films. The fourth part of the films shows the Guillotine, the High Chair, the Large Barrel as well as exercises with the Baby Chair.[2]

Most reports about the Arm Chair stem from teachers that have studied under Romana Kryzanowska, such as MeJo Wiggin or Kathi Ross Nash. They reveal that Romana Kryzanowska's Arm Chair was mostly used by elderly ladies, which is how it earned the nickname "old woman's chair". People with generally weaker upper body strength often used it.

The springs of the traditional Arm Chair are placed a little towards the back and connected to the backrest of the Arm Chair. The backrest is movable and follows the forward movement of the user. Thus, if one shifts one's center of gravity towards the front, the springs and the backrest follow, thereby keeping the spring tension on the same level during the entire movement.

Typical for Pilates, the coordinative training of the muscles, i.e. the interaction of several muscles, is very important. Due to the light springs, the muscles are contracted on the opposite side of the base of the spring. The goal is to improve the functional stabilization of the joints.

Since the shoulder joint is mostly stabilized by muscle, the joint health and prevention depend on the balance and proper interaction of the muscles.

---

[1] Esperanza Aparicio & Javier Pérez: „Hubertus Joseph Pilates - The Biography", (2013), p. 520
[2] Esperanza Aparicio & Javier Pérez: „Hubertus Joseph Pilates - The Biography", (2013), p. 667

Generally, there are two types of Arm Chairs. On the one hand, some try to recreate an exact copy of the Arm Chair used in the studio of Joseph Pilates; on the other hand, some have developed the Chair further in some way.

While the springs of the traditional Arm Chair are usually not replaced, the modern versions of the Arm Chair offer this option and can thus be really challenging for healthy, strong people as well.

Some manufacturers offer another new feature for the traditional Arm Chair: the backward inclined seat surface can be adjusted to a horizontal position with one move, which is very comfortable feature that makes it unnecessary to have a wedge cushion or the like at hand for the sideways knee positions.

Manufacturers of the "traditional" Arm Chairs

- Basil (headquartered in the US) http://www.pilatesdesignsbybasil.com/

- Gratz (headquartered in the US) http://www.pilates-gratz.com/

- PURIST Pilates (headquartered in the UK) http://www.puristpilates.co.uk/

- Pilates Equipment Scandinavia (headquartered in Sweden) http://pilatesequipmentscandinavia.com/

- Scoop Pilates Equipment (headquartered in Portugal) http://scooppilates.pt/

- Tirado Pilates Apparatus (headquartered in the US) http://shop.pilatesapparatus.com/main.sc

- TechnoPilates (headquartered in Italy) http://www.tecnopilates.it/pilates-equipment/eng/

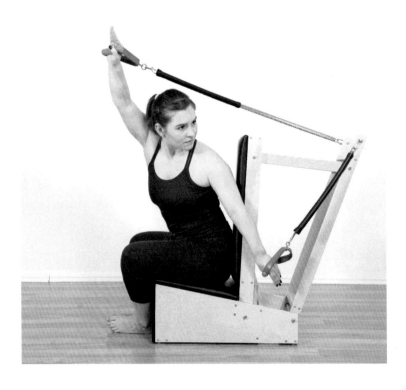

Companies that sell further developed Arm Chairs

- Balanced Body (headquartered in the US) http://www.pilates.com

- BASI Systems (headquartered in Turkey) http://www.basisystems.com/

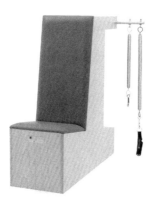 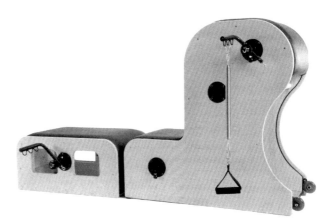

Photos courtesy of Balanced Body

The pictures above show two Arm Chairs from Balanced Body. The left one reminds us of a traditional Arm Chair, but without the movable backrest and with a higher front edge of the seat. Furthermore, it offers the possibility of connecting two pairs of springs of different strength to the device because the metal rod fixes to the back on both sides. Due to the slightly broader fixing, the angle of the energy comes more from the outside. Thus, it is always necessary to slightly work towards the inside while the origin of the spring energy of the "traditional" Arm Chair is more or less parallel to the shoulders.

The right Chair is the so-called Avalon® Arm Chair from Balanced Body, which was created in cooperation with the BASI Pilates® founder Rael Isacowitz. Due to its rotatable lever, which can be attached on many different levels, it offers the possibility to vary the energy origin and intensity of the spring. As shown in the picture below, it can also be used as a Barrel thanks to its slightly rounded surface on the top. Additionally, the optional Box makes it even more versatile so that it can be used, for instance, as a small Wall Unit/Tower, too, as shown in the pictures below.

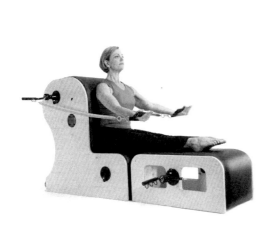 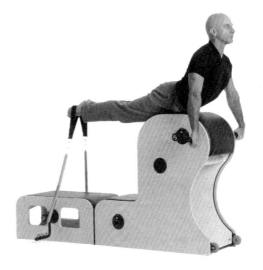

Photos courtesy of Balanced Body

Meanwhile, Rael Isacowitz has created his own equipment line with BASI Systems, which is similar to the Avalon® line from Balanced Body. Pictured below is the Arm Chair Barrel Set. As one can see, a Ladder was added behind the Barrel (this was available at Avalon® as a Ladder Barrel Conversion Kit) and the curvature on the top was increased so that the left side can be used as a complete Ladder Barrel. The curvature can be reduced by using the so-called Arm Chair Saddle, so that it creates a straighter surface like with the Avalon®.

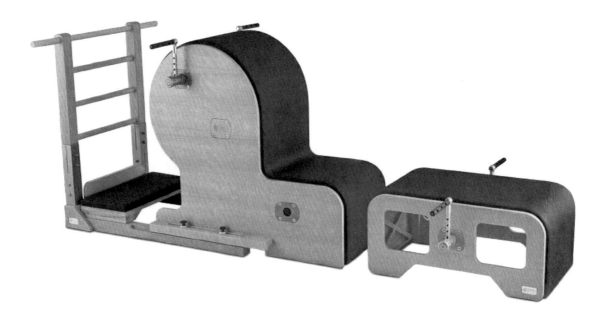

Photo courtesy of BASI Systems; www.basisystems.com; Arm Chair Barrel Set

The Avalon and the BASI Systems Arm Chair Barrel Set both share the feature that the seating position is completely upright, while the traditional Arm Chair and the "regular" Balanced Body Arm Chairs have a slightly backward inclined backrest. Even though this detail seems so minor, it makes all the difference and the necessary amount of work in the stomach to remain flat against the backrest is significantly higher.

Needless to say, the different manufactures use different springs. For the rather "traditional" Arm Chairs very light springs are used; however, one should not underestimate them.

The more modern versions offer different spring lengths and tensions that can be used for different purposes, such as leg work or hip work. One then lies down in front of the Chair or with the Avalon® / BASI versions on top of the Chair and the Box.

Since the hands perform most of the work on the Arm Chair, the connection from the springs to the hands is crucial. Traditionally, one uses either handles with leather loops (left picture) or handles made from aluminum (middle picture). The advantage of the leather loops is that they are relatively soft and do not cut into the hands. Today, the other traditional version, the handles with aluminum loops, is often covered with transparent rubber. However, as these handles tend to cut into the skin despite of the soft transparent rubber coat, they are often covered with a "sheepskin cover" as well (middle picture, right handle).

The modern handle versions are mostly delivered as so-called "neoprene handles" (right picture). They are very flexible and on a par with the other versions even though they are much more affordable.

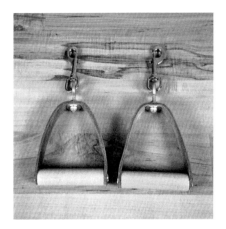 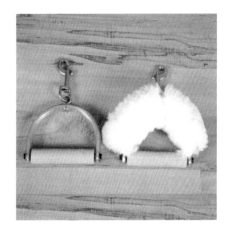 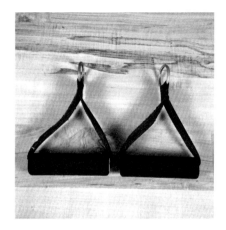

If aluminum handles are used, their weight alone can be enough to wear out the light springs of the traditional Arm Chair. As a precaution, one should therefore hang each spring with the handle side over the opposite end of the device, as recommended by Regina Arras from Top Gun Pilates Engineering Equipment.

Due to the design of the traditional Arm Chair, its springs have contact relatively often with the forearms. Some people do not mind this but others, especially those who are more sensitive, will probably enjoy the so-called sleeves for the springs. These are attached in the front to the handles, stay close to the arms for the entire time when working with the springs and do not shift.

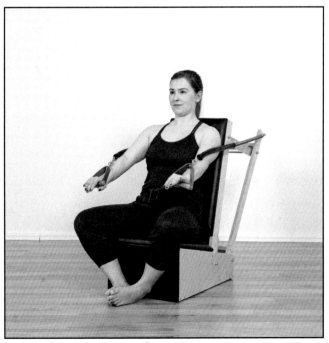

Use of the manual

While the names for the exercises on the mat, the Reformer and the Wunda Chair are relatively consistent in the Pilates world, this is only partly the case for the Arm Chair.

Since the springs on the traditional Arm Chair are not replaced and most exercises presented in this manual refer to the traditional execution of the exercises, there will be no description of the spring tension. If you are using a modern Arm Chair, I suggest adjusting the spring tension to your client in such a way that no compensatory patterns develop and that the already dominant arm and shoulder muscles are not excessively trained to the disadvantage of the other muscles.

Traditional and modern

The traditional Arm Chair repertoire, as it is presented by the students of Romana Kryzanowska, is marked with a (T) for "traditional" behind the exercise, while the exercises that were added at a later time are marked with an (M) for "modern".

Besides the pictures, the descriptions offer access and instructions for each exercise. The following elements are always described:

1. Setup of the exercise
2. Aims of the exercise
3. Execution
4. Common mistakes
5. Modifications or variations

Generally, we have described every step of each exercise, even at the risk of repeating ourselves, so that one can open the page to any exercise at any time and find a full description of it.

In the following, I will give a few notes on the individual description elements.

1. Setup of the exercise

Here we describe the starting position of the exercise. The exercise will only be successful if the starting position is properly adopted. As a first step, it is important to enter a comfortable position and to mentally prepare oneself for the upcoming pattern of movement. If no comfortable position can be found, taking a look at the "variations" can sometimes be helpful. Yet, if no good starting position can be found even after trying alternative positions, you should skip this exercise for the time being.

2. Aims of the exercise

As is known, Joseph Pilates himself always avoided questions about the purpose of single exercises and answered with, "It's good for the body."[1] The latest fasciae research affirms his idea of the body being such a tight network that it has to be considered and trained holistically if possible. For those wanting to know more about the connection between Pilates and fasciae, I recommend the article "Pilates and fascia: The art of 'working in'"by Marie-José Blom.[2]

[1] Ph. D. Peter Fiasca: „Discovering Pure Classical Pilates", (2009), p 47

[2] R. Schleip, T.W. Findley, L. Chaitow, P.A. Huijing: The Tensional Network of the Human Body - The science and clinical applications in manual and movement therapy, (2012), p 449 ff.

Although Joseph Pilates did not articulate aims of an exercise, he was able to give very clear feedback about the desired intention of an exercise via tactile instruction. Unfortunately, one cannot pass on tactile information on paper; hence we describe which muscle groups are targeted and what one is thereby supposed to feel. By this, we also try to narrow down the effect of an exercise and what part of the body it strengthens. The exercise aims can also serve as a means for orientation whether it is suitable at the moment or not.

Furthermore, a pattern of movement can often be performed in different ways. Our body is almost a genius in intuitively avoiding movements that are unfamiliar or strain us and in performing a similar movement pattern by using evasive movement and already strong muscle. By taking a close look at the aims of an exercise, you can try to better detect your evasive tendencies.

3. Execution

Here we initially suggest the number of repetitions. Traditionally, Pilates exercises are often performed with a low number of repetitions. Unfortunately, the time for the setup of some exercises and the time for the actual execution of the exercises are disproportionate. Hence, 4-5 repetitions more are sometimes recommendable. The stated number of repetitions is only a suggestion; depending on the development of the client, one should deviate from this number either towards a higher or lower number. In case of an obvious deficit of one muscle group, one should work in sets, i.e. you repeat an exercise for example five times and after a brief pause you perform two further sets. However, the number of repetitions should never be so high as that the repetitions are executed unfocused or distractedly.

The description of the execution tries to show all necessary steps to successfully execute the exercise. Language is always ambiguous to some extent and we might use other terms than you are used to form your own Pilates experience. Please try to understand and place the terms we use within your own understanding of the movement first.

If there seems to be a contradiction between the pictures of an exercise and the description of the exercise, for instance because the text mentions a straight back but the picture shows a not perfectly upright back, then the text is the point of reference and guides you in the right direction.

4. Common mistakes

Common mistakes are in a way the downside of the aims of the exercise. Here Reiner Grootenhuis reports about his experience with evasive patterns he often observes. Of course, this is only a small selection and it is advisable to always observe your clients closely if they evade a movement and why. If you observe other common mistakes during the exercises in your classes that are not mentioned here, we look forward to your feedback and will add them to later versions.

5. Modifications or variations

Kathy Grant, a master teacher who learnt directly from Joseph Pilates, once said: "I don't do variations. I do applications." With this in mind, variations are not about fighting arising boredom but about adjusting the exercises to the needs of the student if necessary and useful. Sometimes it is merely about making an exercise easier or even harder.

A general rule that Reiner Grootenhuis adopted from Kathy Corey says: "Change the exercises so they fit the people. Find the movement that suits the body."

Exercise positions on the Arm Chair

On the "traditional" Arm Chair, different sitting and kneeling positions are adopted.

1. Sitting, back against the backrest, legs in diamond shape

2. Sitting, back is <u>straight</u> and leaning away from the backrest towards the front

3. Sitting, back is <u>rounded</u> and bent away from the backrest towards the front

4. Kneeling towards the backrest, knees touch the backrest, <u>hips lean against the backrest</u>

5. Kneeling towards the backrest, knees touch the backrest, hips do <u>not</u> lean against the backrest

6. Kneeling towards the backrest, knees placed in the <u>middle</u> of the seat cushion

7. Kneeling with the backrest behind the back and the feet placed on the sides of the Chair

8. Kneeling sideways, leaning against backrest

9. Kneeling sideways, <u>not</u> leaning against backrest

"Modern" sitting positions that were later added.

10. Sitting, back against the backrest, <u>feet flat on the floor</u>

11. Sitting facing backwards with the backrest in front of the chest

12. Sitting sideways

Description of the individual positions:

1. Sitting, back against the backrest, legs in diamond shape

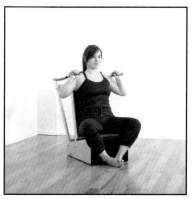

Buttocks, pelvis and lower back are positioned as closely to the backrest as possible while leaning forward, then slowly roll up against the backrest. While doing so, you should be able to feel each vertebra against the backrest and your back should be completely flat without tilting the pelvis posteriorly ("tucked") because of this. The head follows the alignment of the spine and leans against an imagined extended backrest. Consider the alignment of the "box" (see glossary). The soles of the feet are placed against each other. Meanwhile, watch out for a possible dominance of one foot and correct it continuously. The heels are pulled towards the front of the Chair and constantly press in the Chair. Both these activities activate the inner sides of your thighs. The position of the legs is similar to the leg position of the "Seal" on the mat. This position is well suited for opening the lower back. If the position cannot be adopted due to lacking knee flexion, one can for example use a thicker yoga block in order to extend the front part of the Arm Chair. When using a modern Arm Chair, it may be necessary to put a Moon Box or a yoga block under your feet so that a comfortable diamond position can be adopted.

2. Sitting, back is <u>straight</u> and leaning away from the backrest towards the front

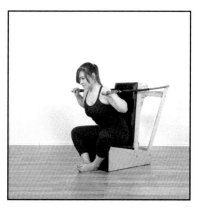

The position of the legs and the feet is identical to the position described under (1). Here the back is slightly tilted forward from the pelvis. The angle will vary from person to person. However, the following applies: the further one leans forward, the harder the position becomes. When using the traditional Arm Chair, the backrest follows the forward motion.
<u>A mixture of position (1) and (2)</u>: The backrest tilts forward and is held against the back only by the strength of the springs. The back is straightened up against the backrest. This variation is not further dealt with in this manual.

3. Sitting, back is <u>rounded</u> and bent away from the backrest towards the front

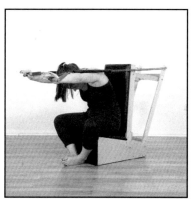

The position of the legs and the feet is identical to the position described under (1). Here the back is rolled forward beginning at the top so that the neck and head are parallel to the floor. The back displays a large C-curve and reminds us of the Spine Stretch.

4. Kneeling towards the backrest, knees touch the backrest, hips lean against the backrest

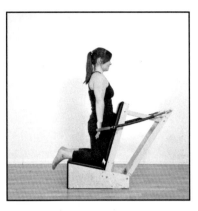

While standing on your knees, the knees are pushed completely against the backrest. Both legs are tightly closed with inner tension. Thighs and hips lean against the backrest, the upper body adopts an erect position. The slight hyperextension from the knees to the hips is not continued upwards.

Thighs, knees and feet are closed and build up tension against each other (inner tension). The feet can either be held in dorsiflexion or plantarflexion. As an alternative, the upper body can also lean diagonally to the front, which engages the back muscles more strongly.

5. Kneeling towards the backrest, knees touch the backrest, hips do not lean against the backrest

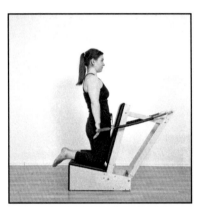

While standing on your knees, the knees are pushed completely against the backrest. Both legs are tightly closed. The upper body adopts an erect position from the knees upwards. Depending on the exercise, one might slightly lean backwards so that on can kneel steadily despite of the spring resistance.

Thighs, knees and feet are closed and build up tension against each other (inner tension). The feet can either be held in dorsiflexion or plantarflexion.

6. Kneeling towards the backrest, knees placed in the <u>middle</u> of the seat cushion

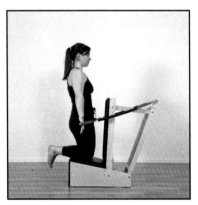

While standing on your knees, place them approximately in the middle of the seat surface. The upper body adopts an erect position from the knees upwards. When using a traditional Arm Chair, the backrest moves towards the person. Due to this a part of the additional spring tension is compensated.

Thighs, knees and feet are closed and build up tension against each other (inner tension). The feet can either be held in dorsiflexion or plantarflexion.

7. Kneeling with the backrest behind the back and the feet placed on the sides of the Chair

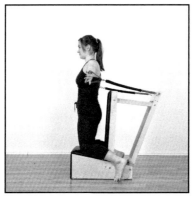

While standing on your knees, position your knees in such a way on the seat surface that the feet can press laterally against the back of the Arm Chair. After building up pressure with the inside of your feet, slowly push your heels together without removing the inner edge of your feet. During this motion, your hip adductors and glutes should be tensed. Straighten up.

When using a modern version of the Arm Chair, it can be difficult adopting this position. If so, perhaps try to do the exercise on a Box in front of the Chair.

8. Kneeling sideways, leaning against the backrest

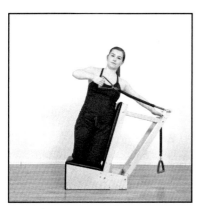

While standing on your knees sideways on the Chair, push your inner knee completely against the backrest. Both legs are tightly closed and build up inner tension. Lean your inner leg (=closer to the base of the spring) and hips against the backrest. The inner arm grabs the transverse frame of the Arm Chair. Pay attention to keeping the body in an erect position and to the "box" (see glossary).

9. Kneeling sideways, not leaning against the backrest

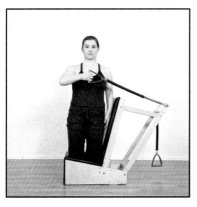

Level the incline of the seat surface of the Arm Chair using a rolled up mat or wedge cushion. Some manufacturers of the traditional Arm Chair also offer a feature to level the seat surface (e.g. Purist Pilates and Edgar Tirado upon request). Stand on your knees sideways on the Chair. Depending on the surface, tightly close your legs and build up inner tension. Straighten up. If you are not using your inner arm, let it hang at your side between your body and the backrest.

10. Sitting, back against the backrest, feet flat on the floor

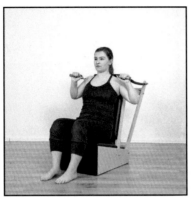

The lower back is positioned as closely to the backrest as possible, then slowly roll up against the backrest. While doing so, you should be able to feel each vertebra against the backrest and your back should be completely flat without tilting the pelvis posteriorly ("tucked") because of this. The head follows the alignment of the spine and leans against an imagined extended backrest. The feet are placed forward in line with the hips in a comfortable distance. The heels continuously press into the ground. The pressure in the forefoot is distributed evenly over the balls of the foot; the arch is lifted.

11. Sitting facing backwards with the backrest in front of the chest

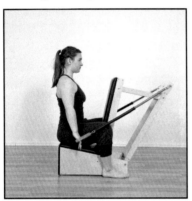

Sit down on the rear edge of the Chair facing the backrest. Your back is in an erect position. The feet are pressed against the sides of the Chair. When using a traditional Arm Chair, one can control the backrest with the knees so that it does not move closer towards you.

The feet are placed in front of you in a comfortable distance. The heels continuously press into the ground. The pressure in the forefoot is distributed evenly over the balls of the foot; the arch is lifted.

12. Sitting sideways

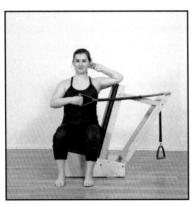

Sit down sideways on the seat surface. In order to sit up straight, perhaps level the seat surface with a wedge cushion.

Your feet are placed forward in line with the hips in a comfortable distance. The heels continuously press into the ground. The pressure in the forefoot is distributed evenly over the balls of the foot; the arch is lifted.

The arm that is closest to the backrest is either placed on the backrest (see picture) or, if this is uncomfortable, besides the body with the hand on the navel.

Assistance

The Arm Chair presents some ideal conditions for instructors that facilitate assisting their clients immensely.

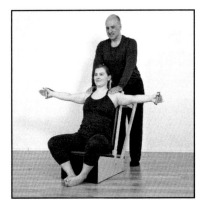

For instance, during the sitting position (1), the instructor can stand behind the Arm Chair and observe how the shoulders behave during the first sitting position (sitting, back against the backrest). If the shoulders, for example, become detached during the Arm Circles, one can hold the shoulders from the top with both hands (fingertips showing to the front) and hence help the shoulders to lean back and stay in contact with the backrest..

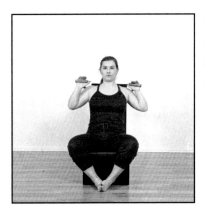

When watching a person from the front during an exercise performed in sitting position (1), as long as the waist is not broader than the backrest one can observe whether the person tilts to the right or to the left. This is especially helpful when training with scoliosis patients.

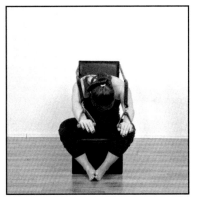

When a person rolls forward on the Arm Chair, one can often observe that they do not roll down in a straight line but tilt to either side. This is well observable information that can initiate a search for the cause of the sideways movement. Certainly, a correction is possible but this rarely remedies the cause.

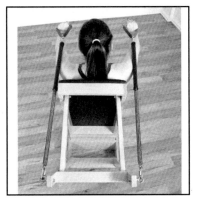

When watching a person while they are performing exercises and when observing the space between the springs and the struts that run from the base of the springs towards the front to the backrest, one is able to detect any laterality very well.

The Arm Chair exercises

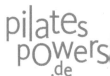

1. Boxing (T)

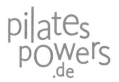

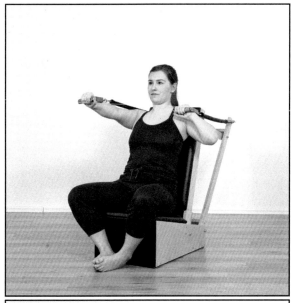

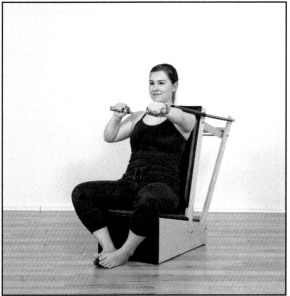

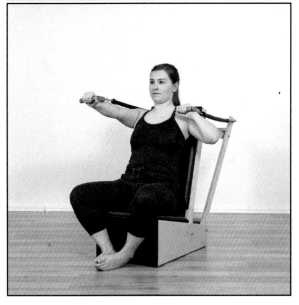

Setup of the exercise:
Position 1. Sitting, back against the backrest, legs in diamond shape. Hands hold the handles with the loops across the top of their wrists. Hands are held at shoulder height. The elbows face outwards.

Aims of the exercise:
Warm up the shoulders
Stabilization: shoulders
Elongation of the torso against the backrest
Strengthening: pectoralis major pars clavicularis and sternalis, anterior part of the deltoid muscle, triceps

Execution : 5x per side
One arm moves forward at shoulder height or slightly above. It is in line with shoulder width or slightly wider but not less wide. While moving the arm backward, the other arm stretches forward. The pace is natural, not like a punch but not too slow as in slow motion either.

Common mistakes:
The shoulder detaches from the backrest every time the arm moves forward.

Modifications or variations:
Position 10. Sitting, back against the backrest, feet flat on the floor

2. Small Arm Circles (T)

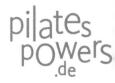

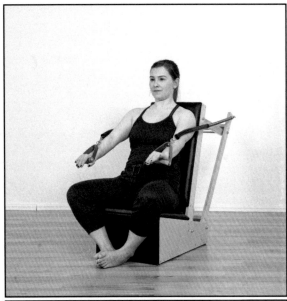

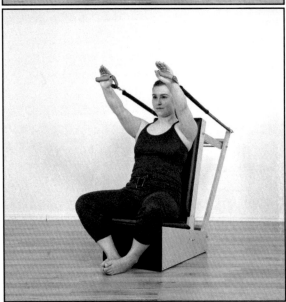

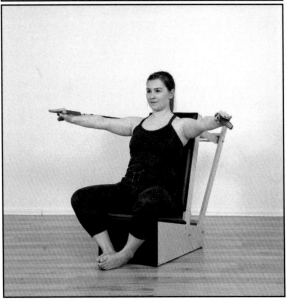

Setup of the exercise:
Position 1. Sitting, back against the backrest, legs in diamond shape. Hands hold the handles with the loops across the top of their wrists. Hands are held at shoulder height.

Aims of the exercise:
Warm up of the shoulders
Stabilization: shoulders
Coordinative training of the anterior muscles stabilizing the shoulder

Execution : 5x in each direction
At a little more than shoulder width apart, stretch both arms forward, the palms face the ground. First lower the arms, then move them outwards and then lift them towards shoulder height. Come back to the starting position. The palms always face towards the ground. Repeat five times, then change direction. The circles should be performed so wide that the hands always remain within your peripheral vision when looking straight ahead with your eyes. Although the exercise is called "Circles" they are actually more semicircles since the top down movement in the first direction is performed in a straight line.

Common mistakes:
The shoulders already round off to the front during the initial phase.

Modifications or variations:
If you experience shoulder pain, perform smaller circles.
Position 10. Sitting, back against the backrest, feet flat on the floor.

3. Hug Sitting Back (T)

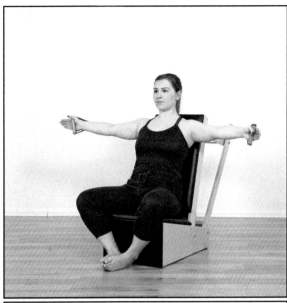

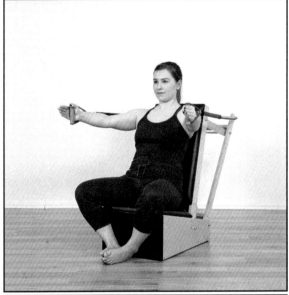

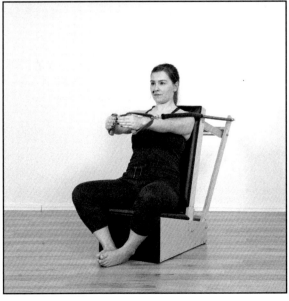

Setup of the exercise:
Position 1. Sitting, back against the backrest, legs in diamond shape. Hands hold the handles with the loops across the top of their wrists. Both arms are opened outward; the hands still remain in front of the shoulders.

Aims of the exercise:
Strengthening: pectoralis major
Training of the muscles controlling the shoulder blades

Execution : 5x
Bring your arms forward together. The elbows are very slightly bent. The hands meet with their fingertips before the arms move back into the starting position again.

Common mistakes:
The shoulders round off while moving the arms forward, the chest slumps down and shoulder blade stability is lost. The connection to the ribs through the external abdominal muscles is lost while moving the arms outwards again.

Modifications or variations:
Position 10. Sitting, back against the backrest, feet flat on the floor.
If the shoulders tend to round off towards the front, only move the arms together until one reaches shoulder width.

4. Boxing Forward Prep (M)

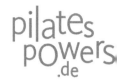
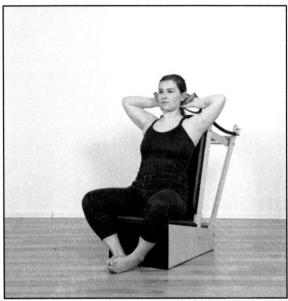

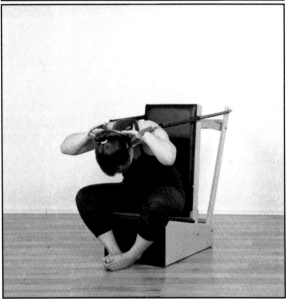

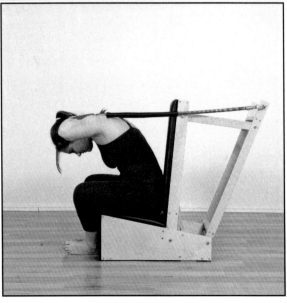

Setup of the exercise:

Position 1. Sitting, back against the backrest, legs in diamond shape. Hands hold the handles with the loops across the top of their wrists. The fingertips of the index and middle finger press against the same fingers on the other hand. The hands are placed behind the head. The elbows are as wide open as possible.

Aims of the exercise:

Preparation for all exercises performed in "Position 3. Sitting, back is rounded and bent away from the backrest towards the front"
Light ab workout
Mobilization: lumbar spine/thoracic spine with a stretching of the long back extensor muscles

Execution : 5x

Starting at the top of the backrest, roll down vertebra by vertebra until a large "C-curve" (see glossary) is reached. Keep the cervical spine elongated while rolling down. Do not rest the chin on your chest. Head and upper back create a long line on which one could place a tray. Imagining rolling over a ball can help achieve the desired form. Then roll up vertebra by vertebra again.

Common mistakes:

Rolling back up is not performed vertebra by vertebra.

Modifications or variations:

Position 10. Sitting, back against the backrest, feet flat on the floor.

5. Hug with Chest Lift (T)

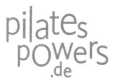

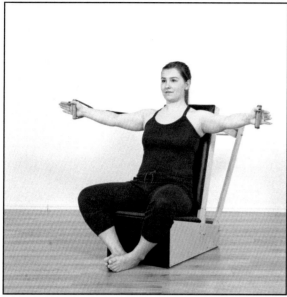

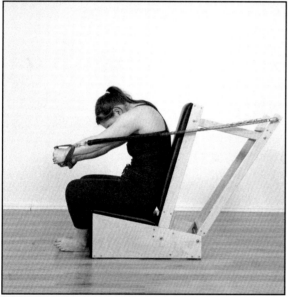

Alternative perspective

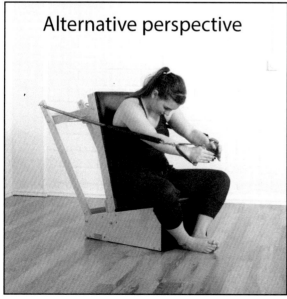

Setup of the exercise:

Position 1. Sitting, back against the backrest, legs in diamond shape. Hands hold the handles with the loops across the top of their wrists. Both arms are opened outward; the hands still remain in front of the shoulders.

Aims of the exercise:

Stabilization of the shoulders despite flexion of the torso
Strengthening: pectoralis major, abdominal muscles
Mobilization: thoracic spine

Execution : 5x

Bring your arms forward together. The elbows are very slightly bent. The hands meet with their fingertips.
At the same time, roll top down until only the tips of the shoulder blades are still touching the backrest. The lower back stays against the backrest. Build up and hold a centered position.
While rolling back vertebra by vertebra, move the arms outwards again.

Common mistakes:

The "Chest Lift" part of the movement is performed too much from the head and not enough by "tilting" beneath the ribs. Passive leaning against the springs instead of active work of the abdominal muscles.
The shoulders round off when stretching the arms forward.
The connection to the ribs through the external abdominal muscles is lost while moving the arms outwards again.

Modifications or variations:

Position 10. Sitting, back against the backrest, feet flat on the floor.
If the shoulders tend to round off towards the front, only move the arms together until shoulder width is reached.

6. Hug Rounding Forward (T)

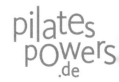
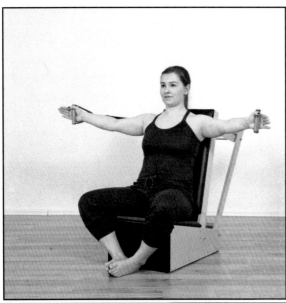

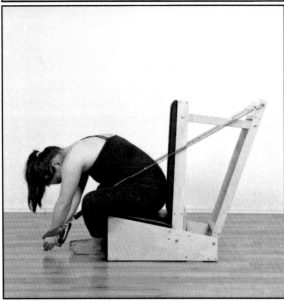

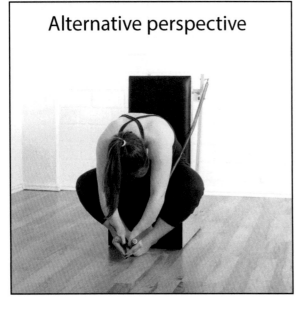

Alternative perspective

Setup of the exercise:
Position 1. Sitting, back against the backrest, legs in diamond shape. Hands hold the handles with the loops across the top of their wrists. Both arms are opened outward, the hands still remain in front of the shoulders.

Aims of the exercise:
Stabilization of the shoulders despite flexion of the torso
Stabilization of the shoulders despite flexion of the torso
Mobilization: lumbar spine/thoracic spine with a stretching of the long back extensor muscles

Execution : 5x
Starting at the top, roll forward as far as possible. The backrest follows the upper body.
Simultaneously, bring your arms forward together. The elbows are very slightly bent. The hands meet with the fingertips.
While rolling back vertebra by vertebra, move the arms outward again. The motion of rolling up vertebra by vertebra is supported by the transversus abdominis and the backrest is slowly guided back up in a controlled manner.

Common mistakes:
Passive leaning against the springs instead of active work of the abdominal muscles.
The shoulders round off when stretching the arms forward.
The connection to the ribs through the external abdominal muscles is lost while moving the arms outward again.

Modifications or variations:
Instead of moving the arms forward simultaneously, first round off to the front and then move the arms together in the Hug.
Position 10. Sitting, back against the backrest, feet flat on the floor.
If the shoulders tend to round off towards the front, only move the arms together until one reaches shoulder width.

7. Kneeling Hug (T)

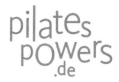
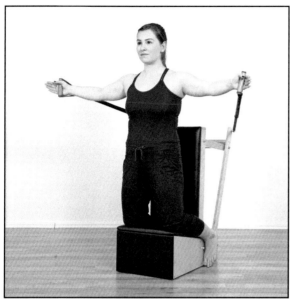

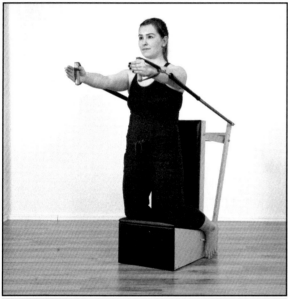

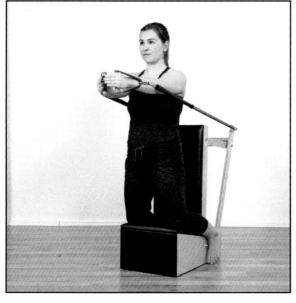

Setup of the exercise:
Position 7. Kneeling with the backrest behind the back and the feet placed on the sides of the Chair. Both arms are opened outward, the hands still remain in front of the shoulders.

Aims of the exercise:
Stabilization: shoulders and torso
Strengthening: pectoralis major (higher spring tension in comparison to the prior seated Hug = higher training effect).

Execution : 5x
Bring your arms forward together. The elbows are very slightly bent. The hands meet with their fingertips before the arms move back into the starting position again.

Common mistakes:
The shoulders round off while moving the arms forward, the chest slumps down and shoulder blade stability is lost. The connection to the ribs through the external abdominal muscles is lost while moving the arms outward again.

Modifications or variations:
If the shoulders tend to round off towards the front, only move the arms together until one reaches shoulder width.
If the exercise cannot be executed well on a modern Arm Chair, perhaps try performing it on a Long Box in front of the Chair. Balance out the distance with the use of respective springs and spring settings.

8. Small Arm Circle with Supination (M)

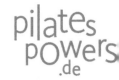

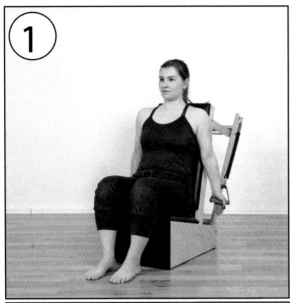

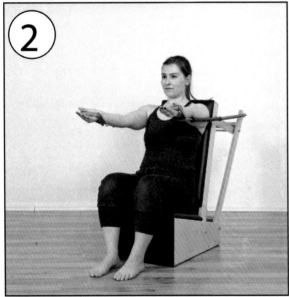

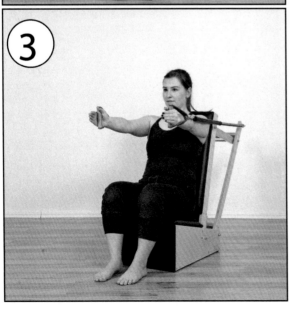

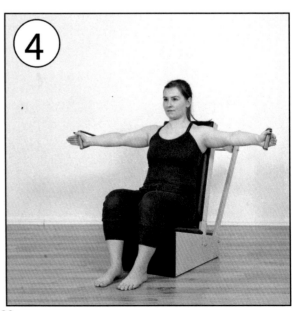

Setup of the exercise:
Position 10. Sitting, back against the backrest, feet flat on the floor. Hands hang laterally at the sides of the body and hold the handles.

Aims of the exercise:
Stabilization: shoulders
Coordinative training of the shoulder stabilizing muscles
Strengthening: pectoralis major, supinator muscles of the forearms and infraspinatus, anterior deltoid muscle and biceps

Execution : 5x in each direction
Lift the arms until shoulder height is reached. Having reached this position, rotate the arms inward so that the palms face each other. Guide the arms outward and from there laterally towards the ground. Change of direction: Lift the arms until shoulder height is reached, move the arms forward until they are at shoulder width ("Hug"). Turn the palms so that they face up and then lower the arms again.

Common mistakes:
Neglecting the inner rotation when lifting the arms. Hold the maximum inner rotation of the arms!

Modifications or variations: -

9. Big Arm Circles (T)

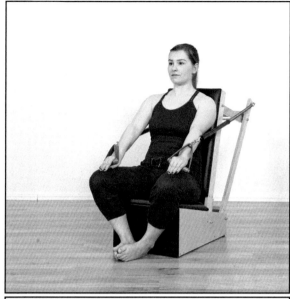

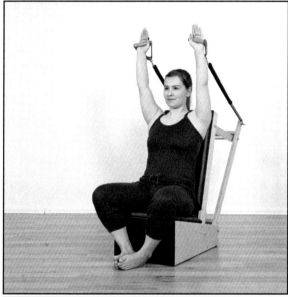

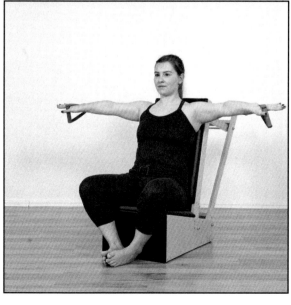

Setup of the exercise:
Position 1. Sitting, back against the backrest, legs in diamond shape. Hands hold the handles with the loops across the top of their wrists. Hands are at shoulder height.

Aims of the exercise:
Improving the range of motion in the shoulders
Stabilization: muscles moving the shoulders
Strengthening: pectoralis major, deltoid muscle
Light strengthening of the latissimus dorsi when moving the arm from its uppermost position to shoulder height

Execution : 5x in each direction
Direction 1: Stretch the arms forward with the palms facing down. First, lower the arms and then move them outward. The palms constantly face down or forward when they are up. Repeat five times, then change direction. Perform the circles as wide as possible. Here too, the circles are rather semicircles as the movement through the "middle" is performed in a straight line

Common mistakes:
The shoulders already round off during the initial phase.
When the arms point up, the shoulders are also lifted.
The upper back detaches from the backrest when over 90 degrees.

Modifications or variations:
Turning the hands at shoulder height so that the palms face up while lowering the arms from the top to the bottom during direction 1.
Lifting the hands with the palms facing up (water scoop) during opposite direction and turning the palms to face down at shoulder height.
Position 10. Sitting, back against the backrest, feet flat on the floor.

10. Kneeling Arm Circles (T)

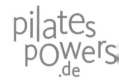
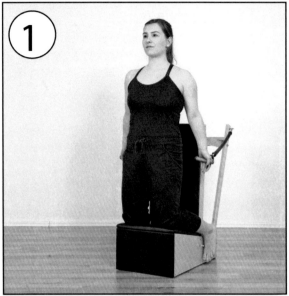

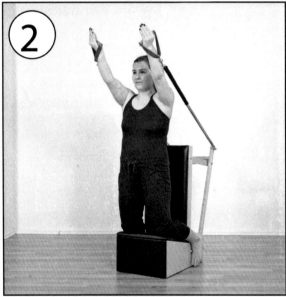

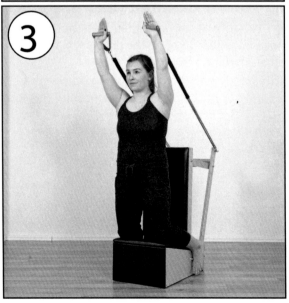

Setup of the exercise:
Position 7. Kneeling with the backrest behind the back and the feet placed on the sides of the Chair.

Aims of the exercise:
Improving the range of motion in the shoulders
Stabilization: shoulders
Stabilization: shoulders
Strengthening: deltoid muscle, pectoralis major, infraspinatus, biceps

Execution : 5x in each direction
Direction 1: Lift the arms together to the top with the palms facing up. At the highest point, turn the palms to face forward. Guide the arms outward and from there laterally towards the ground, the palms face forward.
Repeat five times, then change direction. Perform the circles as wide as possible.
Here too, the circles are more like semicircles as the movement through the "middle" is performed in a straight line.

Common mistakes:
The shoulders already round off during the initial phase.
When the arms point up, the shoulders are also lifted.

Modifications or variations: -

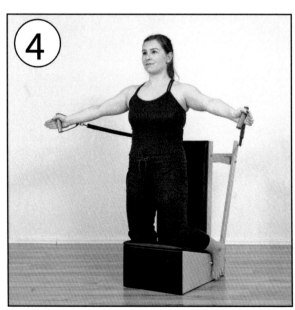

11. Boxing Forward (T)

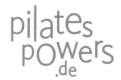

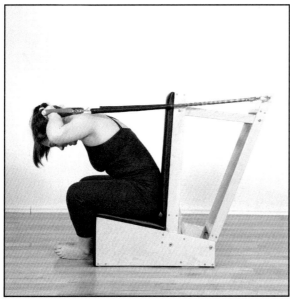

Setup of the exercise:
Position 3. Sitting, back is rounded and bent away from the backrest towards the front. Hands hold the handles with the loops across the top of their wrists. Hands are at shoulder height.

Aims of the exercise:
Stabilization: shoulders
Strengthening: deltoid muscle, triceps, all abdominal muscle groups
Stretching of the back

Execution : 5x per side
One arm is moved forward at shoulder height and parallel to the ground. While this arm is moved backward, the other arm is moved forward.

Common mistakes:
The shoulders lose their stability and move towards the ears.
The upper body swings from side to side during the boxing motion.
The arms are pulled outward.

Modifications or variations:
Position 10. Sitting, back against the backrest, feet flat on the floor.

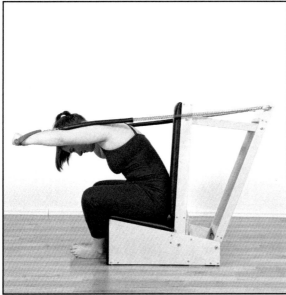

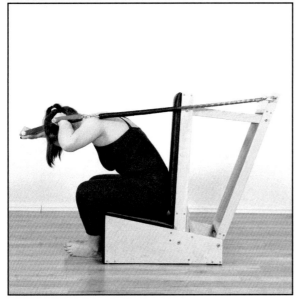

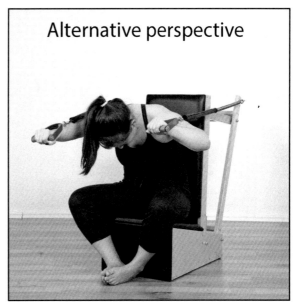

Alternative perspective

12. Boxing Forward & Kick (M)

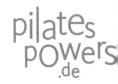
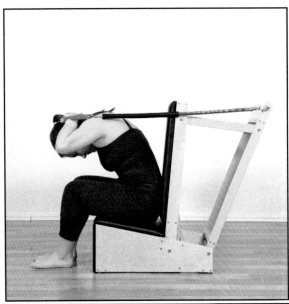

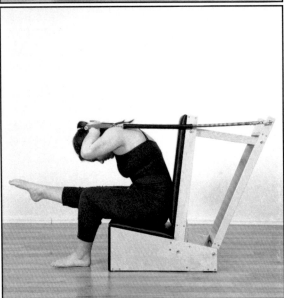

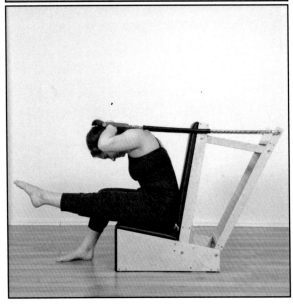

Setup of the exercise:

Position 10. Sitting, back against the backrest, feet flat on the floor. Feet and knees are placed tightly together, inner tension. Hands hold the handles with the loops across the top of their wrists. Shaving position: the fingertips of the thumb and the index finger press against the same fingers on the other hand. The hands are placed behind the head. The elbows are wide. Beginning at the top of the backrest, you roll down to the knees vertebra by vertebra.

Aims of the exercise:

Strengthening: iliopsoas, quadriceps femoris (especially rectus femoris)
Stretching of the back

Execution : 5x per side

While flexing the foot and elongating it by pressing through the heel, extend the foot until it is parallel to the ground. Knees are parallel. Once the extended foot is lifted, it should adopt a pointed position/perform plantar flexion before moving it back to the ground in a large circle. Then change foot.

Common mistakes:

The position of the upper body becomes increasingly upright.
The stretching of the leg is performed in such a way that the knee joint is "compressed." The inner tension is lost when extending the leg.
The knees are not at the same height.

Modifications or variations:

Same exercise but with extended arms. The exercise is then started with already extended arms. At the bottom, the extended arms are parallel to the ground.
Same exercise, like the first variation but one rolls up and down again after every repetition with both legs.

13. Boxing Forward & Kick & Pulses (M)

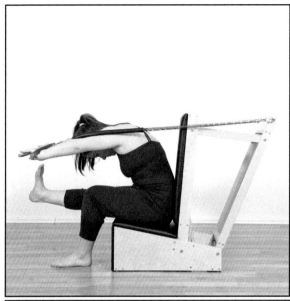

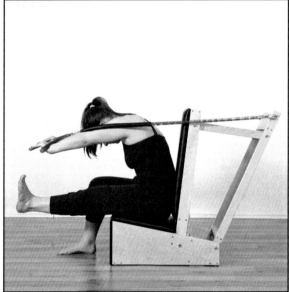

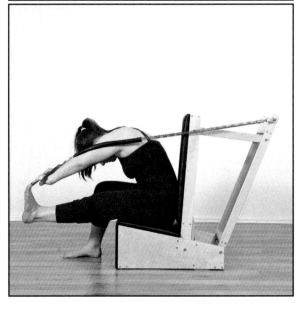

Setup of the exercise:

Position 10. Sitting, back against the backrest, feet flat on the floor.
Feet are placed tightly together.
Hands hold the handles with the loops across the top of their wrists. Shaving position: the fingertips of the thumb and the index finger press against the same fingers on the other hand. The hands are placed behind the head. The elbows are wide. Beginning at the top of the backrest, you roll down to the knees vertebra by vertebra. Extend the arms; fingers keep touching each other.

Aims of the exercise:

Strengthening: hip flexor, quadriceps femoris (especially vastus medialis), light ab workout
Stretching of the back

Execution : 5x per side

While flexing the foot and elongating it by pressing through the heel, extend the foot until it is parallel to the ground. Knees are parallel. Turn the lifted leg outward. Hold plantar flexion in the foot. Perform five pulses towards the ground with the upper body. Place foot back on the ground, change sides.

Common mistakes:

The position of the upper body becomes increasingly upright.
The stretching of the leg is performed in such a way that the knee joint is "compressed".
The pulses derive from the arms.
Only the head nods instead of the upper body pulsing.
The arms are lowered but not the upper body.

Modifications or variations:

Same exercise but instead of performing pulses with the upper body downward, perform 10 pulses with the leg upward.

14. Sparklers (T)

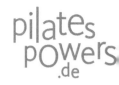

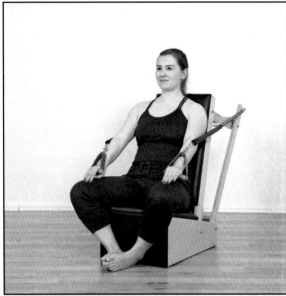

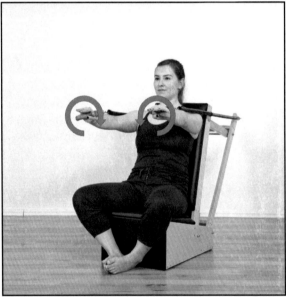

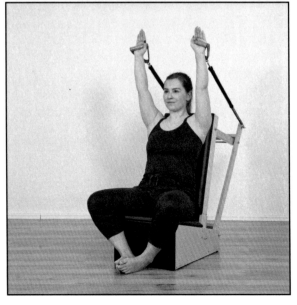

Setup of the exercise:
Position 1. Sitting, back against the backrest, legs in diamond shape. Hands hold the handles with the loops across the top of their wrists.
Hands are at shoulder height.

Aims of the exercise:
Stabilization: shoulders
Coordinative training of the muscles stabilizing the shoulders

Execution :
Small, quick circles as though one were drawing small circles of light with sparklers. Start slightly above the height of your thighs. While performing little circles, move the arms up until they cannot be lifted any further without lifting the shoulders as well. Circle back down and up again. Change the direction of the circles once you reach the top and circle back down, up and down again.

Common mistakes:
Arms are not circled quickly and strongly enough.

Modifications or variations:
Position 2. Sitting, back is straight and leaning away from the backrest towards the front.
Position 10. Sitting, back against the backrest, feet flat on the floor.

15. Chest Expansion (T)

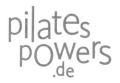

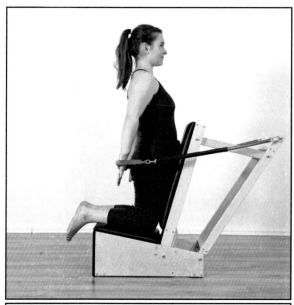

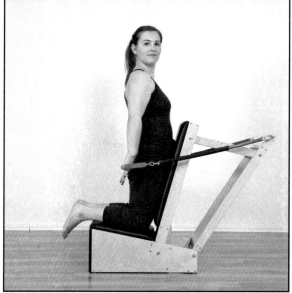

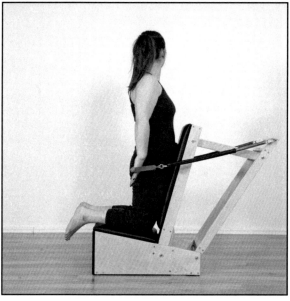

Setup of the exercise:
Position 4. Kneeling towards the backrest, knees touch the backrest, hips lean against the backrest.

Aims of the exercise:
Strengthening: latissimus dorsi, triceps and posterior part of the deltoid muscle
Light stretching of the anterior deltoid muscle
Stabilization: torso by strengthening the long back extensors and the glutes
Mobility: cervical and upper thoracic spine

Execution : 5x
Pull back the arms at the sides of the body. First, turn the head to the right, then to the left and then to the middle. Only then guide the arms back until the springs are relaxed. During the entire movement, keep the shoulders wide open and the torso aligned. In order to optimize the rotation of the head, the shoulder adductors have to be engaged and the shoulder abductors should be as relaxed as possible.

Common mistakes:
The upper body slumps down and the shoulders are pulled forward while the arms are rotated inward. In this case, turning one's head is rather counterproductive.
The head is not turned at the same level but the chin drops during the rotation.

Modifications or variations:
The arm is guided behind the body. From there, one performs small pulses. One starts with 1 pulse and guides the arm back completely; then 1, 2 pulses and guide the arm back; then 1, 2, 3 pulses and back; then 1, 2, 3, 4 - and so on until one reaches the maximum of 10 pulses. And vice versa: 1, 2, 3, 4, 5, 6, 7, 8, 9 and back; 1, 2, 3, 4, 5, 6, 7, 8 and back, etc.
More difficult: Position 5. Kneeling towards the backrest, knees touch the backrest, hips do not lean against the backrest.
Most difficult: Position 6. Kneeling towards the backrest, knees placed in the middle of the seat cushion.

16. Triceps Push Out (M)

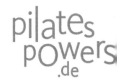

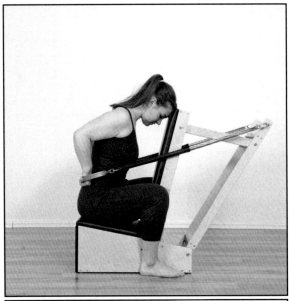

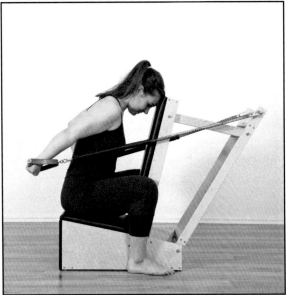

Setup of the exercise:
Position 11. Sitting facing backwards with the backrest in front of the chest. Head leans against the backrest and fixates it. In the back, pull the shoulder blades together and down.
Place your hands above the hips.
Palms face towards the back. Pull the shoulder blades together.

Aims of the exercise:
Strengthening: triceps
Opening of the shoulders

Execution : 5x per arm
Extend each arm alternately. The elbows stay in the same position. Extend the arm completely.

Common mistakes:
Movements are too jerky.

Modifications or variations:
Position 11 but without leaning the head against the backrest.
Position 4. Kneeling towards the backrest, knees touch the backrest, hips lean against the backrest.
More difficult: Position 5. Kneeling towards the backrest, knees touch the backrest, hips do not lean against the backrest.
More difficult: Place hand up higher.
If one side is weaker than the other, do additional repetitions with one arm.

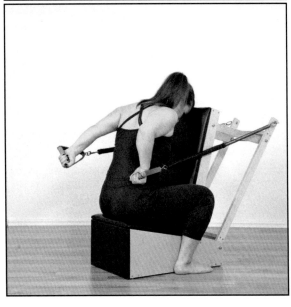

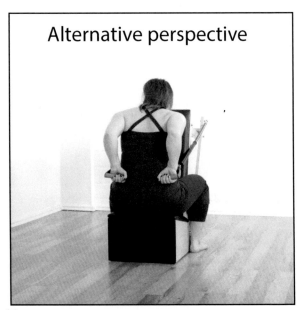

Alternative perspective

17. Kneeling Triceps Push up (T)

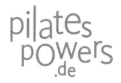

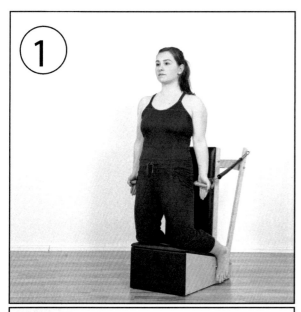

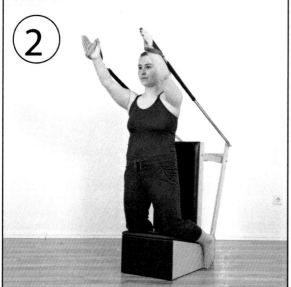

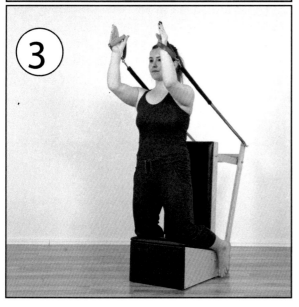

Setup of the exercise:
Position 7. Kneeling with the backrest behind the back and the feet placed on the sides of the Chair.

Aims of the exercise:
Strengthening: triceps
Stabilization: torso and shoulders

Execution : 4x
The extended arms are lifted up at shoulder width apart. Palms face each other. Once the elbows are slightly above shoulder height, the elbows are bent and the forearms are moved back until a 90 degree angle is created. Then extend them again. The elbows stay at the same height. Repeat this four times.

Common mistakes:
Elbows drop while bending the arms and lift while extending the arms. Shoulders are pulled up tightly. Attention: If one leans forward too much, the Arm Chair can tip over.

Modifications or variations:
Easier: Position 1. Sitting, back against the backrest, legs in diamond shape.
Easier: Position 2. Sitting, back is straight and leaning away from the backrest towards the front.

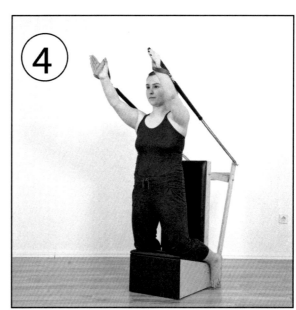

18. Arm Pull Back (T)

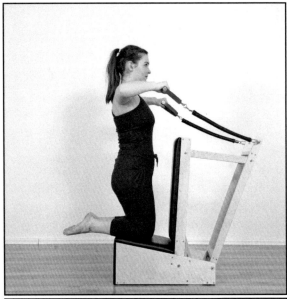

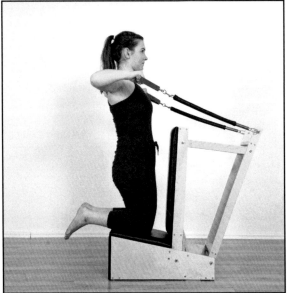

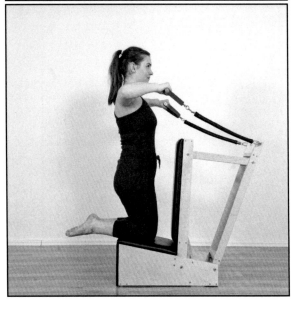

Setup of the exercise:
Position 6. Kneeling towards the backrest, knees placed in the middle of the seat cushion. The back of the Chair moves towards the person during the initial pull. From there keep the springs under constant tension so that the back of the Chair continuously leans towards the person.
Elbows at shoulder height, right angle between forearms and upper arms. Palms face down.

Aims of the exercise:
Strengthening: posterior deltoid muscle, rhomboid muscle

Execution : 5x
Elbows pull back. Simultaneously, the shoulder blades are pulled together. Hold this position for a moment, then release the tension in a controlled manner until the starting position is reached again.

Common mistakes:
The head is pushed forward or overextended towards the back.
The shoulders are pulled up. Elbows or arms drop. The backrest moves during the exercise.

Modifications or variations:
Requires more muscle coordination: Instead of engaging the posterior deltoid muscles and the rhomboid muscles simultaneously, the elbows are first positioned in line with the shoulders by engaging the posterior deltoid muscles. Then the shoulder blades are pulled together. During this process, the elbows do not change their position. Then the shoulder blades are opened again without changing the elbow position and subsequently the elbows are moved forward again.

19. Long Arm Pull Back (M)

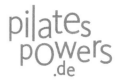

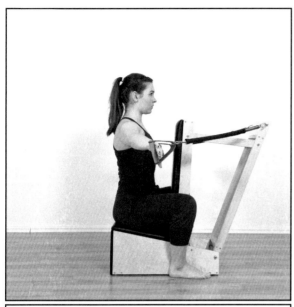

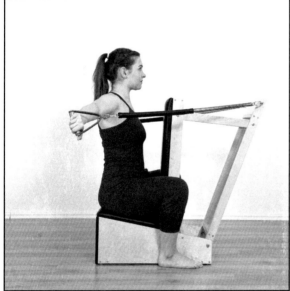

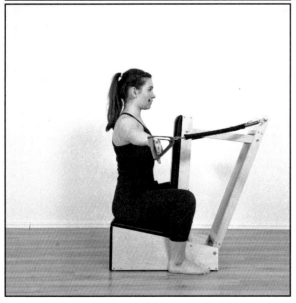

Setup of the exercise:
Position 11. Sitting facing backwards with the backrest in front of the chest. Extend the arms outwards at shoulder height. Turn the palms to the back.

Aims of the exercise:
Strengthening: posterior deltoid muscle, rhomboid muscle, triceps, deltoid muscle (middle part), teres major and subscapularis for the inner rotation at 90° abduction

Execution : 3x sets a 5
Apply tension to the springs and then perform small pulses to the back.

Common mistakes:
The chest bends forward during the small pulses.

Modifications or variations:
Position 5. Kneeling towards the backrest, knees touch the backrest, hips do not lean against the backrest.
Position 6. Kneeling towards the backrest, knees placed in the middle of the seat cushion. The back of the Chair moves towards the person during the initial pull. Keep the springs under constant tension so that the back of the Chair continuously leans towards the person.

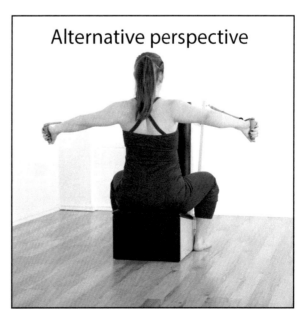

Alternative perspective

20. One Arm Pull (M)

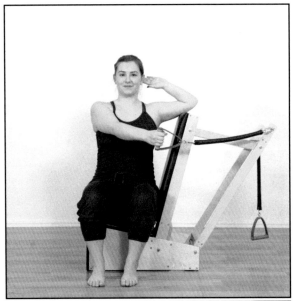

Setup of the exercise:
Position 12. Sitting sideways.
Lift the outer arm forward at shoulder height.

Aims of the exercise:
Strengthening: posterior deltoid muscle
Stabilization: serratus anterior, rhomboid muscle
and triceps

Execution : 5x per arm
Move the extended arm outward in a large curve
until it is in line with the shoulder. This exercise is
very similar to the first exercise of the One Arm
Series (exercise 37) but differs in that the arm is
stiffly moved across the range of motion here, while
the arm slowly unfolds in the Cross Arm Pull
exercise.

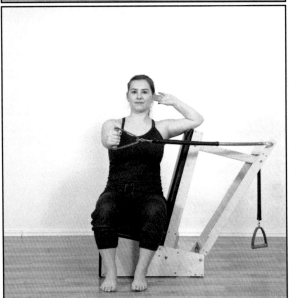

Common mistakes:
The rhomboid muscles pull the shoulder blade
back, thus the posterior deltoid muscle is
strengthened less.

Modifications or variations:
Small pulses at the end of the movement.
If one side is weaker than the other, do additional
repetitions with one arm.

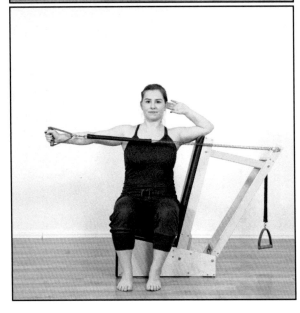

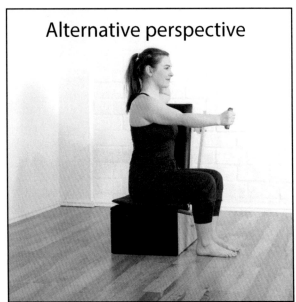

Alternative perspective

21. Cross Arm Rotation (M)

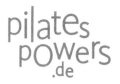

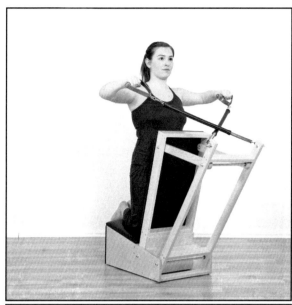

Setup of the exercise:
Position 5. Kneeling towards the backrest, knees touch the backrest, hips do not lean against the backrest.
The springs cross over each other but the hands/arms do not.

Aims of the exercise:
Strengthening: infraspinatus/teres minor and posterior deltoid muscle
Stabilization: serratus anterior, middle deltoid muscle

Execution : 5x
Elbows are at shoulder height. The upper arms form a long line with the shoulders. The forearms create a right angle with the upper arms. This way, the triceps has to be engaged constantly. Imagine a rod running from one elbow to the other. The forearms rotate upwards around this axis.

Common mistakes:
The forearms buckle and decrease the 90 degree angle.

Modifications or variations:
Position 6: Kneel further back: the back of the Chair moves towards the person during the initial pull. From there keep the springs under constant tension so that the back of the Chair continuously leans towards the person.
If one side is weaker than the other, do additional repetitions with one arm.

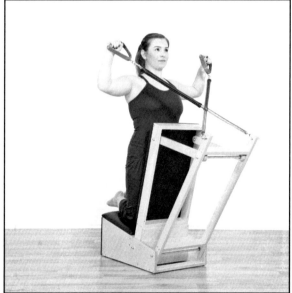

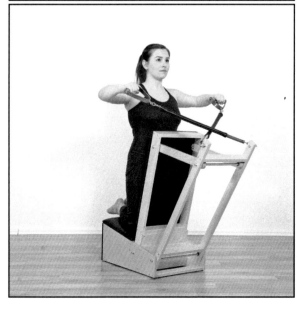

22. Rowing Front from the Chest (T)

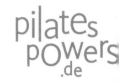

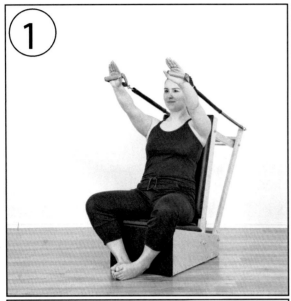

Setup of the exercise:
Position 1. Sitting, back against the backrest, legs in diamond shape. Hands hold the handles with the loops across the top of their wrists. Hands are held at the height of the chest/sternum. Elbows closed.

Aims of the exercise:
Reformer alternative, especially for learning the exercise. Warm up & mobility of the shoulders. Strengthening as for Boxing and Big Arm Circles.

Execution : 3x
Lift both arms up semi-diagonally. From there, lower the extended arms. Move them back to the top position, as far up as possible. Then move the arms outward with the palms facing down. Once they reach the height of the hips, bring the arms back into the starting position.

Common mistakes:
The shoulders lose stability and detach from the backrest.
When the arms are extended upward, the shoulders move towards the ears.

Modifications or variations:
Position 10. Sitting, back against the backrest, feet flat on the floor.

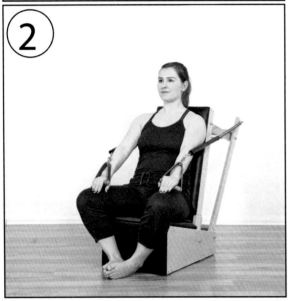

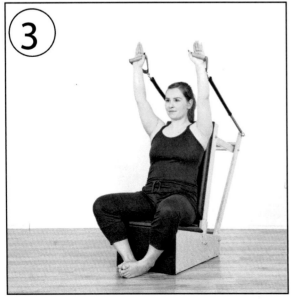

23. Rowing Front from the Hip (T)

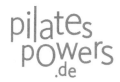

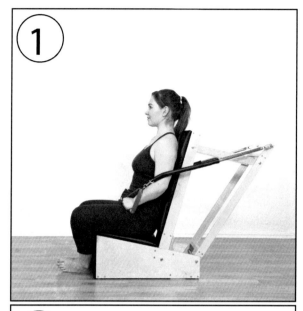

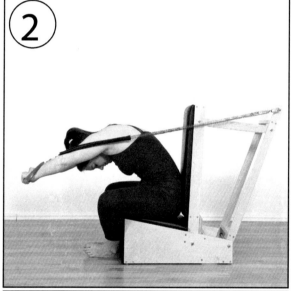

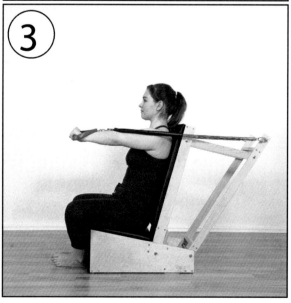

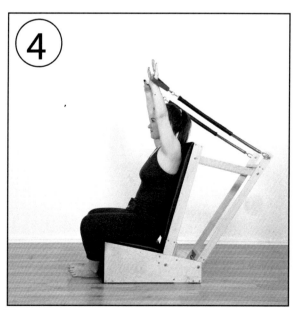

Setup of the exercise:
Position 1. Sitting, back against the backrest, legs in diamond shape. Hands hold the handles with the loops across the top of their wrists. Hands are held slightly above the thighs, elbows closed.

Aims of the exercise:
Reformer alternative, especially for learning the exercise. Warm up & mobility of the shoulders, mobilization of lumbar/thoracic spine with stretching of the long back extensors, control of the horizontal and transverse abdominal muscles.

Execution : 3x
Roll forward in position 3 and extend the arms forward (slightly downward). The backrest also tilts forward. Roll back vertebra by vertebra against the backrest. Arms are parallel to the ground. At the same time, the backrest is gently leaned back. Then move the arms up, outward and down.

Common mistakes:
The shoulders lose stability.

Modifications or variations:
Instead of first leaning completely against the backrest again with the arms parallel to the ground as in picture 3, the movement from picture 2 to picture 4 is performed in one movement.

24. Shaving Sitting Back (T)

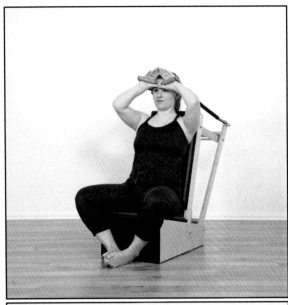

Setup of the exercise:
Position 1. Sitting, back against the backrest, legs in diamond shape. Hands hold the handles with the loops across the top of their wrists. The thumbs and index fingers of both hands press against each other. The hands form a diamond und and are held in front of the forehead. Elbows are wide.

Aims of the exercise:
Stabilization: shoulders
Elongation of the torso against the backrest
Strengthening: triceps and deltoid muscle
stabilized by the serratus anterior

Execution : 5x
Diagonally move the hands up and down along an imagined line.

Common mistakes:
The shoulders lose their stability and move towards the ears.
The thumbs or fingers lose contact.

Modifications or variations:
Position 10. Sitting, back against the backrest, feet flat on the floor.

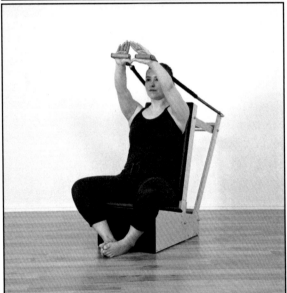

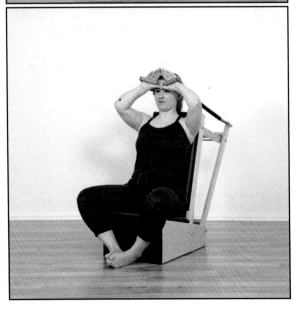

25. Shaving Straight Back (T)

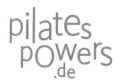

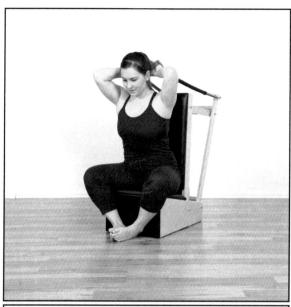

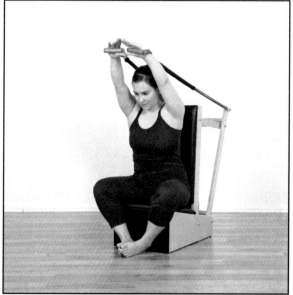

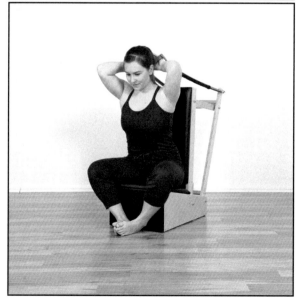

Setup of the exercise:

Position 2. Sitting, back is straight and leaning away from the backrest towards the front. Hands hold the handles with the loops across the top of their wrists.

The thumbs and index fingers of both hands press against each other. The hands form a diamond and are held behind the neck. Elbows are wide.

Aims of the exercise:

Stabilization: shoulders and torso
Strengthening: triceps and deltoid muscle (higher spring tension than for Shaving Sitting Back) stabilized by the serratus anterior

Execution : 5x

Diagonally move the hands up and down along an imagined line.

Common mistakes:

The shoulders lose their stability and move towards the ears.
The thumbs or fingers lose contact.

Modifications or variations:

Position 10. Sitting, back against the backrest, feet flat on the floor.

26. Shaving Forward Round Back (T)

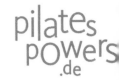

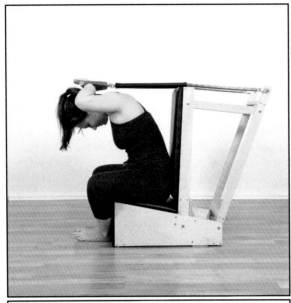

Setup of the exercise:
Position 3. Sitting, back is rounded and bent away from the backrest towards the front. Hands hold the handles with the loops across the top of their wrists.
The thumbs and index fingers of both hands press against each other. The hands form a diamond and are held behind the neck. Elbows are wide.

Aims of the exercise:
Stabilization: shoulders
Strengthening: triceps and deltoid muscle (higher spring tension than for Shaving Straight Back) stabilized by the serratus anterior and all abdominal muscle groups

Execution : 5x
Parallel to the ground, move the hands back and forth along an imagined line.

Common mistakes:
The shoulders lose their stability and move towards the ears.
The thumbs or fingers lose contact.

Modifications or variations:
Position 10. Sitting, back against the backrest, feet flat on the floor.

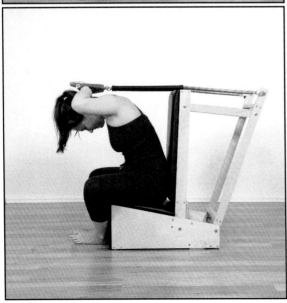

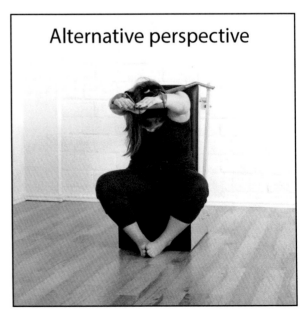

Alternative perspective

27. Kneeling Shaving (T)

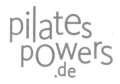

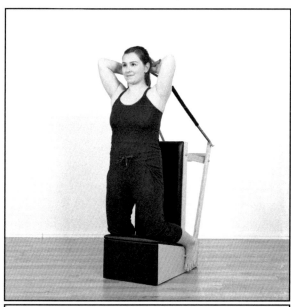

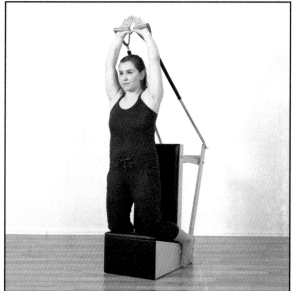

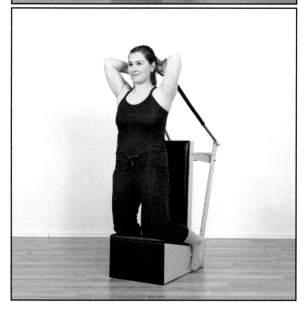

Setup of the exercise:
Position 7. Kneeling with the backrest behind the back and the feet placed on the sides of the Chair. Lift up the arms laterally.
Thumb and index finger press against each other so the hands form a diamond.

Aims of the exercise:
Strengthening: triceps and deltoid muscle
Stabilization: serratus anterior and complete core muscles (coordinative training of the core muscles)

Execution : 3x
Move the hands straight up and down an imagined line. At the end, lower the arms down and outward.

Common mistakes:
The shoulders lose their stability and move towards the ears.
The thumbs or fingers lose contact.

Modifications or variations:
-

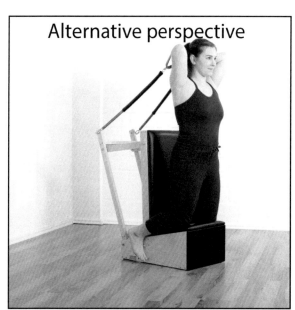

Alternative perspective

28. Swimming Straight Back (M)

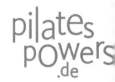

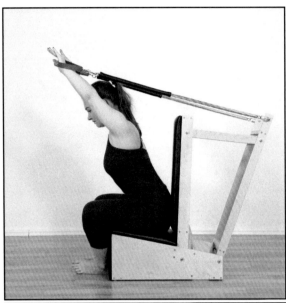

Setup of the exercise:
Position 2. Sitting, back is straight and leaning away from the backrest towards the front. Hands hold the handles with the loops across the top of their wrists.
Arms are stretched as an extension of the spine.

Aims of the exercise:
Mobilization of shoulder joints/blades during maximum elevation with stabilization of the serratus anterior. If elevation ability is limited, strengthening of the deltoid muscle.

Execution : 50x
Arms perform a small up/down swimming stroke.

Common mistakes:
The upper body loses stability and starts swinging.
The shoulders are lifted towards the ears.
The elbows move further apart.
The movement is performed mostly at the end of one's own range of motion making it jerky and less precise.

Modifications or variations:
Position 10. Sitting, back against the backrest, feet flat on the floor.

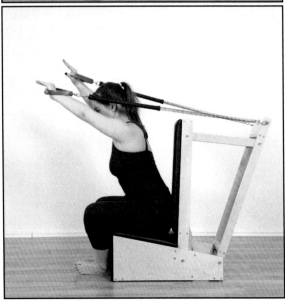

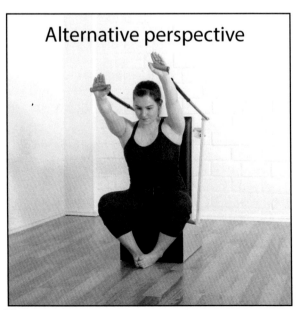

Alternative perspective

29. Side-to-Side (T)

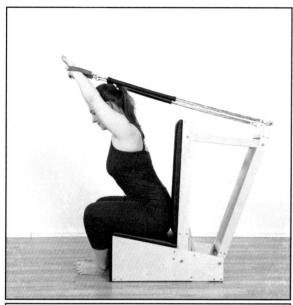

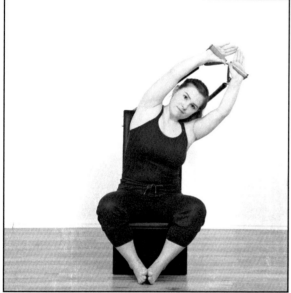

Setup of the exercise:

Position 2. Sitting, back is straight and leaning away from the backrest towards the front. Hands hold the handles with the loops across the top of their wrists.
Lift up the arms laterally. The thumbs and index fingers of both hands press against each other. The hands form a diamond.

Aims of the exercise:

Mobilization: lumbar/thoracic spine.
Strengthening: transverse abdominal muscles
Complete stretching of the respective opposite side including the latissimus

Execution : 3x Sets

First, stretch the upper body beginning at the bottom. Then slightly bend to one side. When performing the movement, there should be equal pressure on both buttocks.

Common mistakes:

Rocking from one buttock to the other.

Modifications or variations:

-

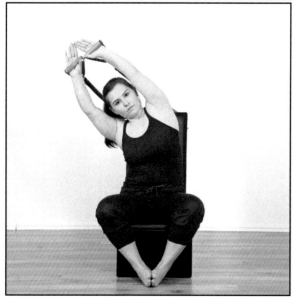

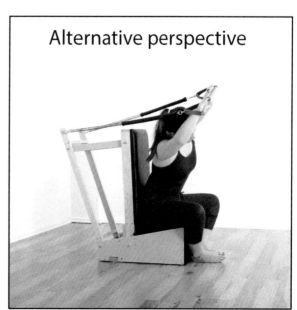

Alternative perspective

30. Butterfly Sitting Back (T)

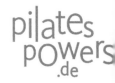

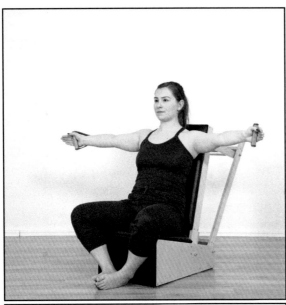

Setup of the exercise:
Position 1. Sitting, back against the backrest, legs in diamond shape. Both arms are opened to the sides as for the "Hug."

Aims of the exercise:
Mobilization of the entire spine while rotating with low resistance
Strengthening: transverse abdominal muscles and deltoid muscle
Coordinative training of the muscles stabilizing the shoulders

Execution : 3x Sets
Beginning at the bottom, the upper body rotates to the right while the pelvis is held steady. During this motion, the right arm is lowered and rotated inward. Simultaneously, the left arm is laterally elevated and the palm faces in the direction of the rotation. Chest and head perform the rotation as well as possible. Come back to starting position. Change side.

Common mistakes:
The shoulder of the elevated arm is lifted.

Modifications or variations:
Position 10. Sitting, back against the backrest, feet flat on the floor.

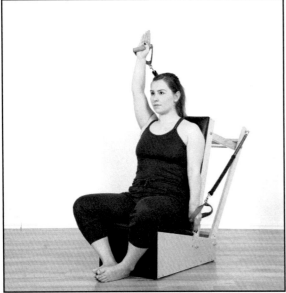

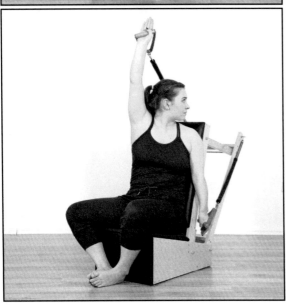

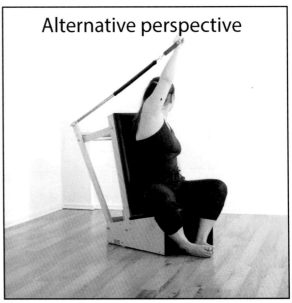

Alternative perspective

31. Butterfly Straight Back (T)

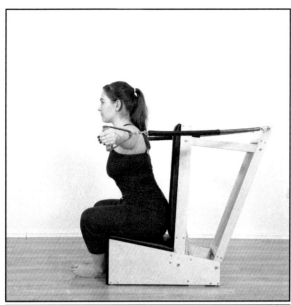

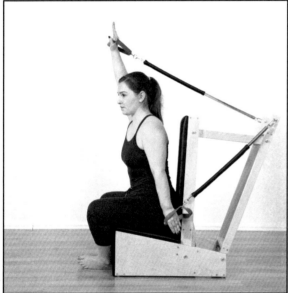

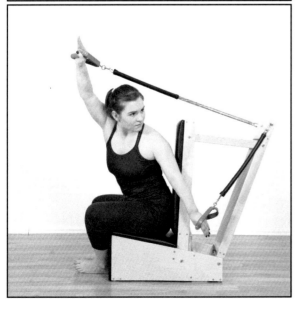

Setup of the exercise:
Position 2. Sitting, back is straight and leaning away from the backrest towards the front. Both arms are opened outward.

Aims of the exercise:
Mobilization of the entire spine while rotating with low resistance, higher mobility than in the previous exercise
Strengthening: transverse abdominal muscles and deltoid muscle
Coordinative training of the muscles stabilizing the shoulders

Execution : 3x Sets
Beginning at the bottom, the upper body rotates to the right while the pelvis is held steady. During this motion, the right arm is lowered and rotated inward. The right palm faces the side of the Arm Chair. Simultaneously, the left arm is laterally elevated and the palm faces in the direction of the rotation. Chest and head perform the rotation as well as possible. Come back to starting position. Change side.

Common mistakes:
The shoulder of the extended arm is lifted.

Modifications or variations:
Position 10. Sitting, feet flat on the floor, but the back is upright and leans forward away from the backrest.

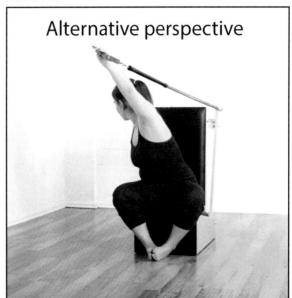

Alternative perspective

32. Kneeling Butterfly (T)

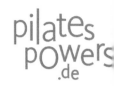

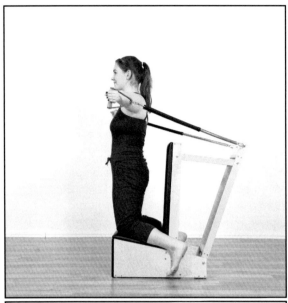

Setup of the exercise:
Position 7. Kneeling with the backrest behind the back and the feet placed on the sides of the Chair.

Aims of the exercise:
Mobilization of the entire spine while rotating with low resistance
Strengthening: transverse abdominal muscles and deltoid muscle
Coordinative training of the muscles stabilizing the shoulders and torso

Execution : 3x Sets
Beginning at the bottom, the upper body rotates to the right while the pelvis is held steady. During this motion, the right arm is lowered and rotated inward. The right palm faces the side of the Arm Chair. Simultaneously, the left arm is laterally elevated and the palm faces in the direction of the rotation. Chest and head perform the rotation as well as possible.
Come back to starting position. Change side.

Common mistakes:
The shoulder of the extended arm is lifted.

Modifications or variations:
-

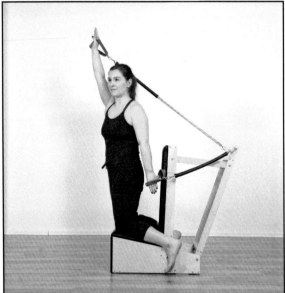

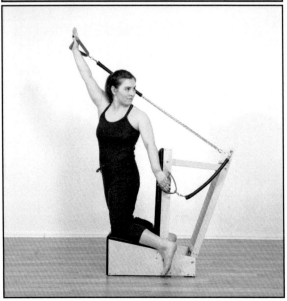

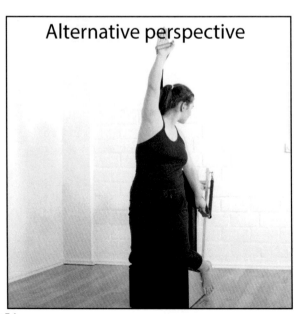

Alternative perspective

33. Spine Twist (T)

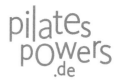

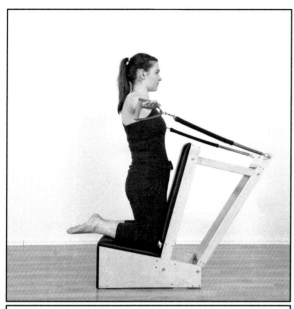

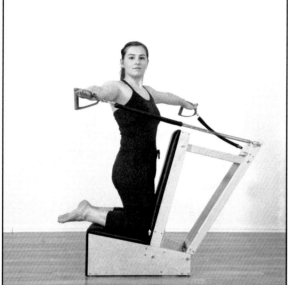

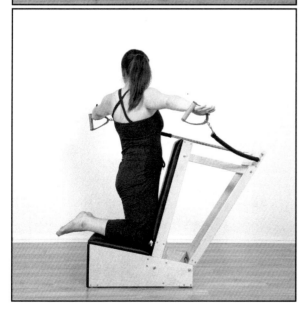

Setup of the exercise:
Position 5. Kneeling towards the backrest, knees touch the backrest, hips do not lean against the backrest. Arms are extended to the sides. Please regard the close-up of the hand below for special instruction on the hand position.

Aims of the exercise:
Strengthening: posterior deltoid muscle, torso rotators
Stabilization: triceps
Coordinative training of the core muscles

Execution : 5x Sets
The movement is similar to the Spine Twist on the mat. Start the rotation of the spine at the hips. Yet, the hips first turn differently than for the same exercise on the mat. Hold the arms steady forming a line and turn them against the resistance of the spring. The head is turned slightly further than the chest. Come back to starting position. Change side.

Common mistakes:
Hips move from side to side. Too much arm movement that exceeds the upper body rotation.

Modifications or variations:
More difficult: Position 6. Kneeling towards the backrest, knees placed in the middle of the seat cushion.

Close-up hand position

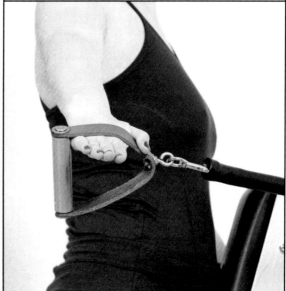

34. Breathing(T)

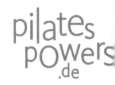
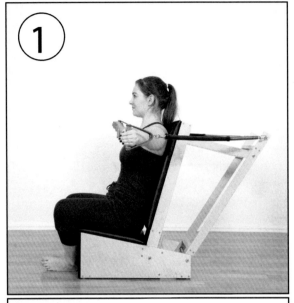

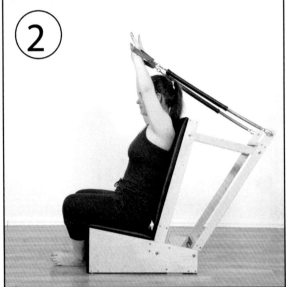

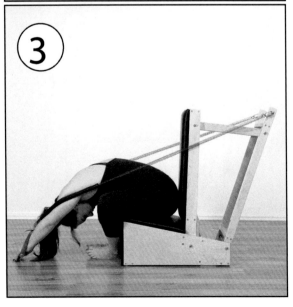

Setup of the exercise:
Position 1. Sitting, back against the backrest, legs in diamond shape. Hands hold the handles with the loops across the top of their wrists.
Arms are wide open.

Aims of the exercise:
Breathing exercise with simultaneous mobilization of the lumbar/thoracic spine and stretching of the long back extensors.

Execution : 3x
First, inhale with the hands to the sides. Then while exhaling, extend the arms slightly broader than shoulder width and roll forward vertebra by vertebra in a large curve. The backrest follows the forward movement. The hands touch the ground as far as possible in front of you, thereby completely deflating the lungs. Then while inhaling, roll back against the backrest vertebra by vertebra, and open the arms to the sides.

Modifications or variations:
-

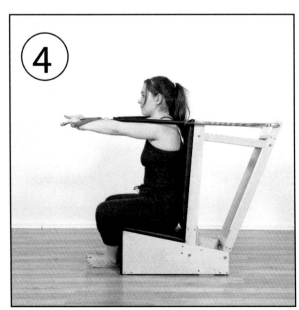

35. Saw (T)

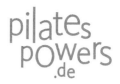

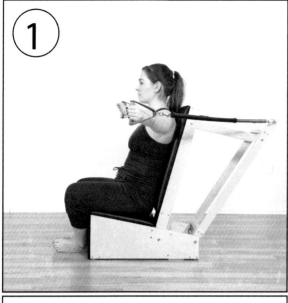

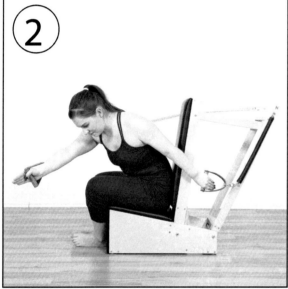

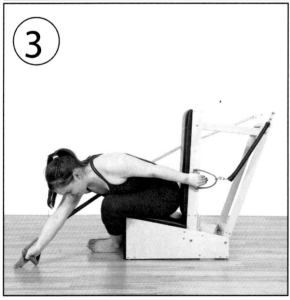

Setup of the exercise:
Position 1. Sitting, back against the backrest, legs in diamond shape. Hands hold the handles with the loops across the top of their wrists.
Arms are wide open.

Aims of the exercise:
Stretching: latissimus
Mobilization: lumbar/thoracic spine with flexion and light rotation
Coordinative training of the core muscles, especially when straightening up

Execution : 3x Sets
The upper body rolls down vertebra by vertebra. The spine rotates slightly and leans across the left thigh. The pelvis is held steady. The left arm pulls back and then up. The left palm faces the side of the Arm Chair. The right arm extends forward diagonally towards the ground. "Reach" forward as far as possible. Move back completely into the starting position before changing sides.

Common mistakes:
Shoulder moves towards the ear.
Exercise is performed jerkily and with too little patience.

Modifications or variations: -

Alternative perspective

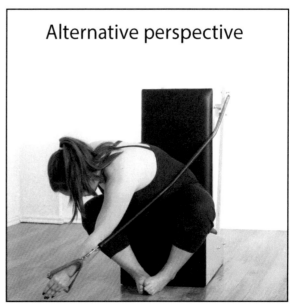

36. Butterfly Swimming (T)

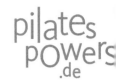

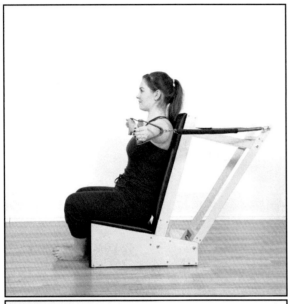

Setup of the exercise:
Position 1. Sitting, back against the backrest, legs in diamond shape. Hands hold the handles with the loops across the top of their wrists.
Arms are wide open.

Aims of the exercise:
Control of asymmetries in the posture, detected through one spring slipping off the backrest towards one side.

Execution : 3x
Move the arms up together and then lower them quickly forward towards the ground. During this motion, lean the upper body forward in a controlled manner. The springs run across the front edge during this exercise. Roll back at the same quick pace and move the arms back into starting position. The breathing pattern is opposite to the pattern in exercise 34 "Breathing." Roll forward while inhaling, roll back while exhaling.

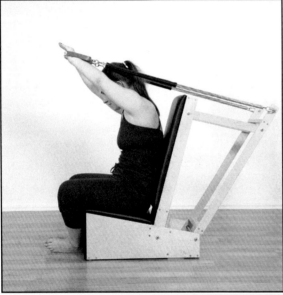

Common mistakes:
The shoulders lose their stability and move towards the ears.

Modifications or variations: -

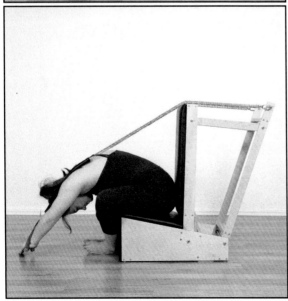

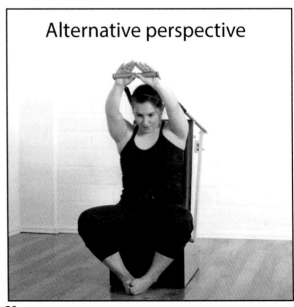

Alternative perspective

37. One Arm Series - Cross Arm Pull (1/6) (T)

Originally called: Swakatee or Swaquity/Swockety/Swakkiti

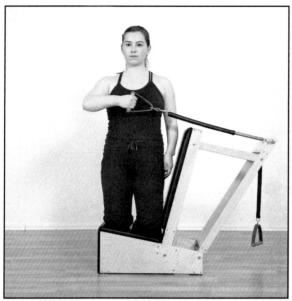

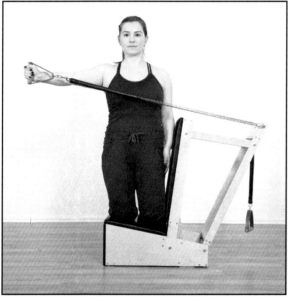

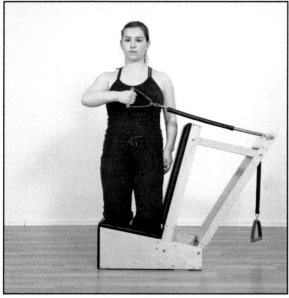

Setup of the exercise:
Position 9. Kneeling sideways, not leaning against backrest. The outer arm is at shoulder height and bent so that the hand is in front of the chest or the opposite shoulder.

Aims of the exercise:
Strengthening: posterior deltoid muscle and triceps while regarding control of the torso

Execution : 4x per side
The outer arm is moved outward in a flowing motion as though one were opening a large door. Similar to a backfist strike. The arm is moved back in the same manner.
Change sides after the fourth repetition.

Common mistakes:
The movement of the arm is divided into two single movements: elbow strike and then extension of the arm. This way, more strain is put on the elbow joint.

Modifications or variations:
Head turns in the direction of the hand during the fourth repetition.
If one does not put a cushion or wedge cushion under the inner knee, best adopt position 8. Kneeling sideways, leaning against backrest.

Alternative hand position

38. Shaving up the side of the head (2/6) (T)

Originally called: Uppa

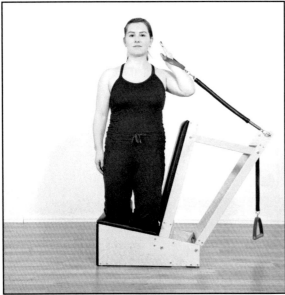

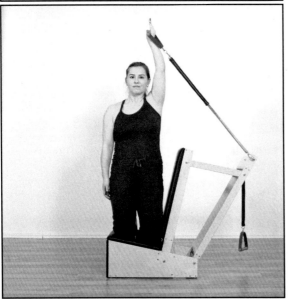

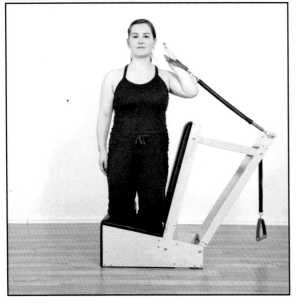

Setup of the exercise:

Position 9. Kneeling sideways, not leaning against backrest. Place the hand of the inner arm at ear height with the elbow facing outward.

Aims of the exercise:

Strengthening: Entire deltoid muscle and triceps while regarding control of the torso

Execution : 4x per side

Extend the arm up in a straight line from the outside of the shoulder until its maximum extension is reached, then lower it back to the ear. Change sides after the fourth repetition.

Common mistakes:

The arm deviates from the "ideal" line towards the side or the front.
The shoulder loses stability and moves towards the ear.

Modifications or variations:

If one does not put a cushion or wedge cushion under the inner knee, best adopt position 8. Kneeling sideways, leaning against backrest.

39. Cross Arm Pull & Shaving (3/6) (T)

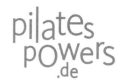

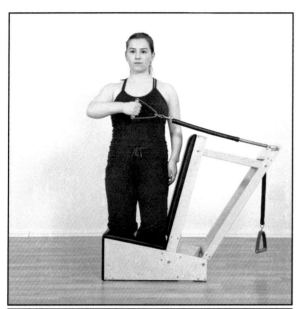

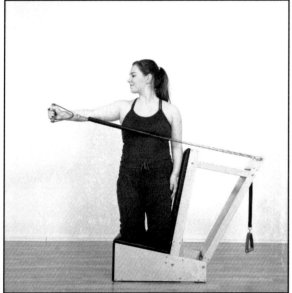

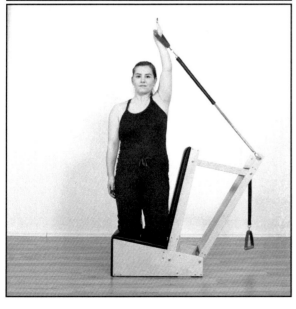

Setup of the exercise:
Position 9. Kneeling sideways, not leaning against backrest.

Aims of the exercise:
Strengthening: deltoid muscle and triceps while regarding control of the torso

Execution : 3x per side
Cross Arm Pull: The outer arm is at shoulder height and bent so that the hand is in front of the chest or the opposite shoulder.
The outer arm is moved outward in a flowing motion as though one were opening a large door. The head follows the motion and turns so that it faces the extended arm. The arm is moved back in the same manner.
Then change hand and arm.
Shaving: extend the arm up in a straight line from the outside of the shoulder until its maximum extension is reached, then lower it back to the ear. Change again.
Change sides after the third repetition of the set.

Common mistakes:
Cross Arm Pull: the movement of the arm is divided into two single movements: elbow strike and then extension of the arm. This way, more strain is put on the elbow joint.
Shaving: the arm deviates from the "ideal" line to the side or the front.
The shoulder loses stability and moves towards the ear.

Modifications or variations:
If one does not put a cushion or wedge cushion under the inner knee, best adopt position 8. Kneeling sideways, leaning against backrest.

40. Triceps/Propeller (4/6) (T)

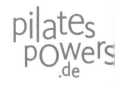

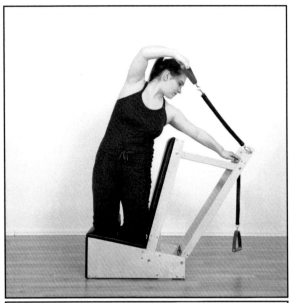

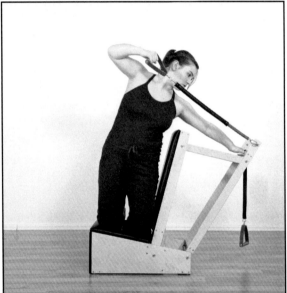

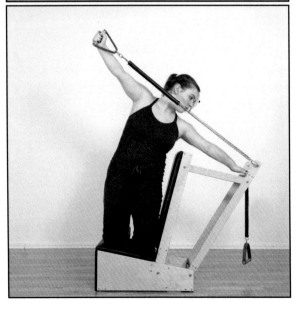

Setup of the exercise:

Position 9. Kneeling sideways, not leaning against backrest, while bending to the side towards the backrest and placing the hand on the transverse bar. Lift up the outer arm, the hand points down and holds the handle of the anterior spring. The elbow is slightly bent. When performing the exercise, the hand should only move as close to the body as there is sufficient distance between the spring and the face.

Aims of the exercise:

Strengthening: triceps
Light stretching: latissimus and transverse abdominal muscles
Light mobilization: lumbar/thoracic spine in lateral flexion

Execution : 4x per side

While remaining in the same position and without changing the height of the elbow, extend the outer arm. Thereby the hand automatically turns so that it faces away from the body. Then bend the arm again to return into starting position. Change sides after the fourth repetition.

Common mistakes:

Elbow of the outer arm moves up and down. This way, the triceps is less engaged.

Modifications or variations:

If one does not put a cushion or wedge cushion under the inner knee, best adopt position 8. Kneeling sideways, leaning against backrest.

41. Circles both ways (5/6) (T)

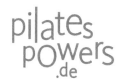

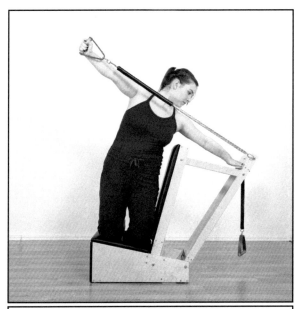

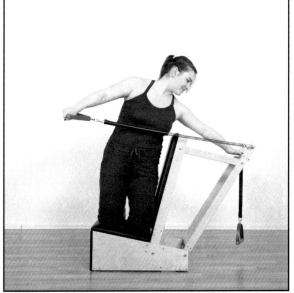

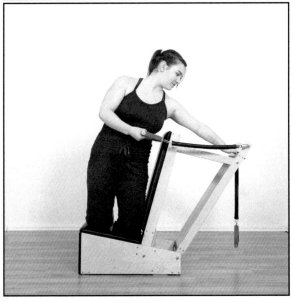

Setup of the exercise:
Position 9. Kneeling sideways, not leaning against backrest, while bending to the side towards the backrest and placing the hand on the transverse bar. Lift up the outer arm, the hand points down and holds the handle of the anterior spring. The elbow is slightly bent. When performing the exercise, the hand should only move as close to the body as there is sufficient distance between the spring and the face.

Aims of the exercise:
Strengthening: triceps, deltoid muscle and supraspinatus
Light stretching: latissimus and transverse abdominal muscles
Light mobilization: lumbar/thoracic spine in lateral flexion
Coordinative training of the shoulder blade muscles

Execution : 3x in both directions per side
Move the outer arm back and downward. The palm faces down at the outermost point. Once the hand reaches the lower part of the radius, the palm faces up.
As soon as the spring loses its tension, the arm and hand are returned into the starting position of exercise 40 Triceps/Propeller.
Change sides after three repetitions in both directions.

Common mistakes:
The range of the movement is not fully used.

Modifications or variations:
If one does not put a cushion or wedge cushion under the inner knee, best adopt position 8. Kneeling sideways, leaning against backrest.

42. Lotus Flower (6/6) (T)

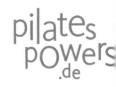

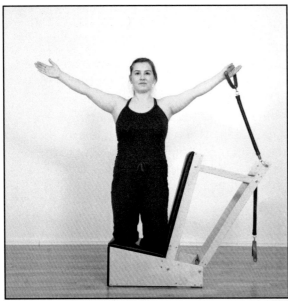

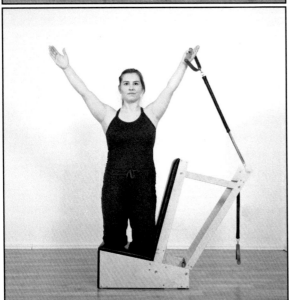

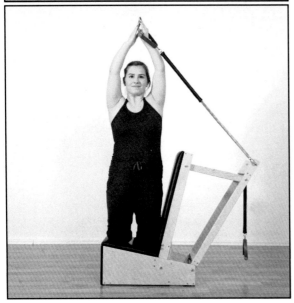

Setup of the exercise:
Position 9. Kneeling sideways, not leaning against backrest. Both hands are extended to the sides and the open palms face up. The hand that is closest to the springs holds the handle of the anterior spring. The spring is put under minimal tension and does not sag.

Aims of the exercise:
Strengthening: deltoid muscle
Stabilization: torso

Execution : 4x per side
Move both arms toward each other with bent elbows. The fingertips of both hands touch. Both arms open to the sides until the starting position is reached again.
Change sides after the fourth repetition.

Common mistakes:
Trying to support the arm, the upper body moves away from the base of the spring.
The moving arm bends more strongly than the relaxed arm in order to facilitate the angle of strength.

Modifications or variations:
If one does not put a cushion or wedge cushion under the inner knee, best adopt position 8. Kneeling sideways, leaning against backrest.

Glossary (1/4)

2 way stretch	A basic principle of Pilates in which one tries to pull the body apart into two directions starting from the body's middle. One direction of movement is the necessary contrast for the other direction of movement. An outer movement is not always visible.
Abdominal	Refers to the abdominal wall and all abdominal muscle groups. This does not yet indicate which group is engaged (also see → Transversus abdominis).
Back extensors	All muscles that are involved in the extension of the back. They are divided into short back extensors (e.g. multifidi) and → long back extensors.
Biceps	More precisely musculus biceps brachii. This muscle bends the arm at the elbow joint and rotates the forearm outwards (strongest supinator). It consists of two parts. It is an antagonist of the musculus triceps brachii.
Box	The box is a concept that helps aligning the body. It represents an imagined line from shoulder to shoulder and hip to hip. Both lines are parallel to each other. Also, there is an imagined line on both sides that runs from the hip to the shoulder, which are parallel to each other as well. Together the four lines form a box. There is another smaller box within this box, which represents the connection between the lower ribs and the bony protrusion of the iliac crest (spina iliaca anterior superior).
C-curve	A recurrent basic form in Pilates, in which the pelvis, spine and head form a large C when viewed from the side. This form can be achieved by adopting a position in which the pelvis is tilted posteriorly (also see → Posterior pelvic tilt), the → transversus abdomini muscle hollows out the abdominal muscles, the ribs flow together, the sternum slightly slumps down and the head is tilted so that it is in line with the spine. Simultaneously, the back is stretched.
Deltoid muscle	The muscle surrounds the shoulder joint and is crucial for lifting the arm. It is divided in an anterior (pars clavicularis), a middle (pars acromialis) and a posterior (pars spinalis) part. Up to 60 degrees abduction, the middle part is mainly engaged; only after this point do the other two parts become abductors as well. Before this, they mainly act as adductors due to their location in relation to the axis of the shoulder joint.
Dorsiflexion	Movement of the foot in the ankle joint towards the shin (opposite: → plantar flexion).
Elevation	Lifting of the arm over the horizontal level (= continuation of the abduction).
Fasciae	Colloquially called connective tissue. More precisely, fasciae are the soft tissue of the connective tissue. Fasciae is a topic that is still being researched. What is special about them is that their role in the body was totally underestimated until roughly 2007 (the date of the first international congress on the topic of fasciae). Today we know that fasciae, for instance, are able to transmit kinetic energy and pain, to name but two.
Glutes	Consist mainly of the muscles gluteus maximus, gluteus medius, gluteus minimus and piriformis. Their main purposes are the extension, outer rotation and abduction of the leg in the hip joint.

Glossary (2/4)

Hip flexor	The hip flexors mainly include the → iliopsoas and the rectus femoris. Yet, various other muscles are also involved like the tensor fasciae latae, sartorius, gracilis and adductor longus and brevis.
Infraspinatus	Part of the rotator cuff, which keeps the humerus head inside its articular cavity. It starts at the fossa infraspinata of the shoulder blade and ends at the tuberculum majus of the humerus. Depending on the position of the shoulder joint, it also helps with the abduction or adduction.
Iliopsoas	The iliopsoas (= hip flexor) consists of the psoas (starting at the lumbar spine) and the iliacus (starting at the inner ilium). Both are attached to the trochanter minor of the femur.
Lateroflexion	Bending to the side.
Latissimus dorsi	Also called broad back muscle. It starts at the lower vertebrae of the thoracic spine and continues until the last lumbar vertebra. From there, it runs across both sides towards the axilla as a flat, broad muscle. It narrows on its way to the axilla and is attached to the humerus near the shoulder joint. Its main function is to pull the arm towards the body and a little towards the back.
Long back extensor	Subgroup of the back extensors. They are also called musculus erector spinae. Essentially, the group consists of the following three parts: musculus iliocostalis, musculus longissimus, and musculus spinalis. The muscles extend over the entire length of the spine laterally beside the spinous process. While the long back extensors are mainly responsible for the overall movements, the short back extensors mostly stabilize and move the individual segments (one vertebra against the other).
Lumbar region	Region of the lumbar spine.
Muscles moving the shoulder blades	The shoulder blade is attached to the thorax by muscles (→ trapezius, → rhomboids, → serratus anterior). In order to lift the upper arm over 90 degrees, these muscles must rotate the shoulder blade so that there is more room under the roof of the shoulder (acromion).
Muscular imbalances	Imbalance between muscles that move a joint. For example, the interaction of biceps and triceps for bending/extending the arm. A muscular imbalance can occur due to too short and too strong biceps. As a result, the arm cannot anymore be extended completely. Such imbalances can be caused by overtraining one side and neglecting the other but also by a lack of physical activity, one-sided daily movements or injuries.
Musculoskeletal system	Collective term for muscles and fasciae.
Myofascial release therapy	Fasciae can, for example, thicken, wrinkle, or stick together and thus affect our mobility and can also cause significant pain. Such fasciae problems can be treated with therapeutic methods like Rolfing or manual therapy based on the Fascial Distortion Model by Typaldos.

Glossary (3/4)

Pectoralis major	The large chest muscle pulls the arm towards the body and rotates it inward. It is divided in pars clavicularis (upper part, is also attached to the clavicle), pars sternalis (middle part, mainly attached to the sternum) and pars abdominalis (lower part).
Plantar flexion	Bending the foot in the upper ankle joint in direction of the sole of the foot or away from the shin (also see dorsiflexion).
Posterior pelvic tilt	The upper edge of the pelvis tilts backward, thereby the pubic bone tilts forward.
Powerhouse	The abdominal and back muscles combined with the pelvic floor and diaphragm form a steady container. All movements are imagined originating from this central point.
Quadriceps femoris	Four-headed knee extensor, which is involved in the hip extension with one of its parts - the musculus rectus femoris.
Rhomboids	Consist of two parallel parts (=musculus rhomboideus major and minor), which, together with other muscles, attach the shoulder blades to the thorax. They move the shoulder blades closer to the spinous process - where they are attached - and cause a slight pull upward. They originate from the medial border of the shoulder blade.
Serratus anterior	Also called the sawing muscle. It connects the shoulder blade with the ribs. It prevents the shoulder blade from uncontrollably lifting off the anterior thorax (the so-called winged scapula) and is the antagonist of the → rhomboids.
Subscapularis	It originates from the side of the shoulder blade that faces the thorax. It's tendon pulls in front of the humerus head and mainly causes an inward rotation of the humerus in the shoulder joint. It is part of the rotator cuff.
Supinators of the forearm	They rotate the forearm in the elbow joint outward so that the palm faces up when the upper arm lies flat against the side of the body and the elbow is bent in a right angle. The → biceps is the strongest supinator. It is supported by the musculus supinator and brachioradialis.
Supraspinatus	Part of the rotator cuff, which holds the humerus head in the articular cavity. The supraspinatus is mainly responsible for beginning the abduction in the shoulder joint before the → deltoid muscle can unfold its strength.
Teres major	Connects the outer inferior angle of the shoulder blade with the humerus and moves them closer together.
Teres minor	The smallest unit of the rotator cuff that mainly causes an outward rotation and adduction in the shoulder joint.
Torso rotators	Rotation of the torso around its own axis.
Transverse abdominal muscles	Consist of the exterior (= musculus obliquus externus abdominis) and the interior (= musculus obliquus internus abdominis) transverse muscles. They can rotate and tilt the upper body on the pelvis and tilt the pelvis backward during co-contraction. Furthermore, they belong to the muscles supporting the breathing as they support exhalation.

Glossary (4/4)

Transversus abdominis — Due to its mainly horizontal orientation, it is best for performing the abdominal press. Also, it supports exhalation.

Trapezius — The trapezius muscle originates at the spinous process of the thoracic and cervical spine and continues upward to the occiput. Depending on its orientation, it is divided into a descending and an ascending region. The entire scapular spine, acromion and outer third serve as a long attachment for this muscle. Depending on which region of the muscle is contracted, it either rotates, adducts, lifts or lowers the shoulder blade.

Triceps — More precisely musculus triceps brachii. Extends the arm in the elbow joint and adducts it in the shoulder joint. It consists of three parts. The → biceps is its strongest antagonist.

Acknowledgements

First of all, I want to thank my wife. When I started to take an interest in Pilates, it became clear very quickly that Pilates was not only going to be a hobby. The endurance she had taking care of our family during the many hours of my education and her patience when I brought home all the Pilates equipment that soon filled an entire room are unforgettable. Only sometimes I tested her patience too much when I scrambled about my Pilates equipment for hours until the middle of the night because one movement did not feel right. The change from being a manager to being the owner and instructor of a Pilates studio was challenging in many ways, too, and would not have been possible without my wife. Thank you!

I dedicate this training manual to my wife and children.

I would also like to thank my first Pilates instructor Mario Alfonso, who endured all of my typical German analytical questions during our lessons. A great challenge for an Italian. Without his help, I would have probably never been able to complete my Pilates education.

I share a special bond with my BASI Pilates teacher Miriam Friedrich Honorio, whose profound understanding of movement and especially of quality of movement has influenced me immensely.

I also thank Alexandra Clasen, whose Gyrotonic Studio is my refuge week after week and with whom I can discuss the topic of movement from a different perspective than from Pilates. A true inspiration.

Special thanks go to the Pilates teachers that have significantly influenced my view on Pilates: Rael Isacowitz, Brett Howard and especially Kathy Corey.

Finally, I want to thank my clients, trainees and instructors at pilates-powers. Without the possibility of exploring, deconstructing and discovering all of the Pilates exercises with different types of bodies anew, this training manual would not exist.

Thank you!

Tönisvorst, September 2016   Reiner Grootenhuis

Literature recommendations

Pilates

Pilates
Author: Rael Isacowitz; publisher: Human Kinetics; 2014 (English); (Kindle Edition available) (second edition)

Pilates Anatomy: Pilates Anatomy: Your illustrated guide to mat work for core stability and balance
Authors: Rael Isacowitz, Karen Clippinger; 2011; (English); (Kindle Edition available)

Pilates an interactive workbook
Author: Christiana Maria Gadar; publisher: Gadar Inc.; 2013; (English)

Einführung in den Wunda Chair
Author: Reiner Grootenhuis; publisher: CreateSpace Independent Publishing Platform; 2015; (German); (Kindle Edition available)

History

Joseph Pilates - Der Mann, dessen Name Programm wurde
Authors: Eva Rincke; publisher: Herder publisher; 2015; (German)

Hubertus Joseph Pilates - The Biography
Authors: Esperanza Aparicio & Javier Pérez; 2013; (English); (iBook Edition available)

About the authors

Reiner Grootenhuis

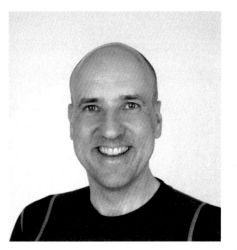

Besides obtaining a diploma in psychology and an MBA, Reiner Grootenhuis has studied the healing and martial arts of the Southern Shaolin Monastery Weng Chun. He completed the training as a Pilates instructor for Pilates mat and equipment at the Pilates educational academy BASI® (Body Arts & Science International). He is the founder and operator of the largest Pilates forum worldwide, pilates-contrology-forum on Facebook, which includes 6,900 Pilates instructors. At the beginning of 2012, he opened the pilates-powers Studio in Tönisvorst. Since 2014, he has been offering his own Pilates education program. In the same year, Kathy Corey appointed him a member of the Board of Directors of the Pilates Heritage Congress, which takes place every two years in the hometown of Joseph Pilates. In 2015, he published the first publicly available German training manual on the Wunda Chair. Since January 2016, he has been studying the finesse of the method within the Kathy Corey mentor program.

Dr. Ingo Barck

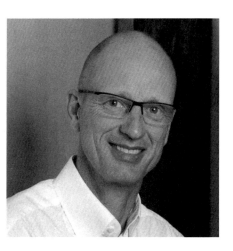

Dr. Ingo Barck has always been a passionate athlete. Over the course of his life, he has performed various sports such as swimming, athletics, rowing, handball, underwater rugby, diving, paragliding, kitesurfing, triathlon, and judo (certified trainer/long-standing work as a trainer). Today he enjoys running, swimming, bicycle racing, inline skating, skiing, wakeboarding and, since 2013, Pilates.

The certified doctor was able to gain experience in orthopedics and surgery as well as some insight in the industry in 2007 before he pursued working as a manual therapist for patients suffering from pain in his own private medical practice. His particular focus is on the connective tissue (fasciae), which has gained increased recognition over the past few years.

Made in the USA
San Bernardino, CA
25 January 2017